A PRESCHOOL HEALTH CURRICULUM

Here We Go... Watch Me Grow!

Charlotte Hendricks, HSD
Connie Jo Smith, EdS

Illustrated by Nic Frising

ETR Associates
Santa Cruz, California 1991

About the Authors

Charlotte Hendricks, HSD, and **Connie Jo Smith, EdS,** bring together years of experience in preschool education. Their training and areas of expertise complement each other.

Hendricks is an assistant professor in the Department of Health Education and Physical Education at the University of Alabama at Birmingham. Smith works with Training and Technical Assistance Services at Western Kentucky University.

Hendricks's years as a health educator in community and university settings blend with Smith's experience as a preschool educator and consultant. Both authors were instrumental in the development of the *Hale and Hardy Helpful Health Hints* preschool health curriculum, which serves as the background for the development of this new curriculum.

© 1991 by ETR Associates. All rights reserved.
Published by ETR Associates,
P.O. Box 1830, Santa Cruz, CA 95061-1830.
To order call toll-free 1-800-321-4407.

Printed in the United States of America

10 9 8 7 6 5 4

Cover design: Julia Chiapella
Text design: Ann Smiley

Title No. 592

Library of Congress Cataloging-in-Publication Data

Hendricks, Charlotte Mitchell, 1957-
    Here we go—watch me grow! : a preschool health curriculum / Charlotte M. Hendricks, Connie Jo Smith ; illustrated by Nic Frising.
      p. cm.
    ISBN 1-56071-048-9
    1. Health education (Preschool)—United States—Curricula—Handbooks, manuals, etc. 2. Teaching—Aids and devices—Handbooks, manuals, etc. 3. Education (Preschool)—United States— Activity programs—Handbooks, manuals, etc. I. Smith, Connie Jo. II. Title.
LB1140.5.H4H46   1991
372.3'7043—dc20   90-23323

Dedication
· · · · · · · · · · · · ·

To my husband, Jim, my parents and my grandmother Gardner.

—CMH

• • •

This book is dedicated to Becky Bennett, who has inspired me to grow toward a healthy lifestyle, and to Breanne Thompson, whom I wish happy and healthy life choices.

—CJS

Contents

Acknowledgments
•••••••••••••••••••••••

The authors would like to express sincere appreciation to the following individuals:

Kathleen Middleton—For her support, encouragement and expertise throughout the development and revision of this curriculum.

David M. Macrina—For his technical review during revision of this curriculum and for helping us create a document that makes sense to the reader.

Becky Bennett—For the many hours spent in search of children's songs, books, poems, rhymes and fingerplays that met our criteria for inclusion in this curriculum.

The authors would also like to thank the following people for their review of materials and their assistance in evaluation of the curriculum:

Jerry Aldridge   Gary Nelson
Diane Allensworth   Clarence Pearson
Millie Cowles   Fred Peterson
Danise Echols   R. Morgan Pigg
Ann Eddowes   Roger Schmidt
Glenn Lohr   Howard Taras
Roberta Long

Introduction

Preschool years are crucial to the development of behaviors that contribute to physical, emotional and social health. Fortunately, preschool is no longer viewed as a time when children are merely watched by professional babysitters. We now realize that we can significantly enhance learning opportunities for young children by providing sound educational experiences. This opportunity for teaching and learning has significant implications for the developing health of the child.

Early education about health can begin a lifelong process of learning about ourselves and our relationships to others and to the world around us. The experiences children have around health and ways to improve it will enhance their desire and ability to make wise decisions. Preschool health education provides a foundation for health education in elementary school and beyond.

This curriculum guide is based on a belief in the potential of health education for preschoolers. It is a response to the scarcity of current health education resources available to preschool teachers. This innovative curriculum is designed to be both academically sound and practical. The activities facilitate learning through hands-on interactive processes between children and their environment.

The curriculum uses an integrated approach to provide for all areas of child development. Health is the primary focus, and the curriculum is structured around units with specific health content themes.

These thematic units parallel the basic subject areas of health education addressed in educational settings beyond preschool. Areas addressed are growth and development, mental and emotional health, personal health, family life and health, nutrition, disease prevention and control, safety and first aid, consumer health, drug use and abuse and community health. The units can be used in sequence over the course of a nine- or twelve-month time frame, or they can be used individually at the teacher's discretion.

Teacher Considerations

Traditional learning centers are an integral component of this curriculum. These centers are areas inside or outside the classroom that are arranged to encourage children to actively explore materials and interact with other children and adults.

Each objective includes suggestions for materials and activities to add to traditional learning centers, such as art, blocks, housekeeping, manipulative (fine motor) and science centers. Special learning centers are also suggested for some objectives.

The basic learning strategies used in this curriculum are fully described in a special section. Each objective includes variations of activities based on these learning strategies. The objectives also include additional activities designed specifically for each objective.

The suggested activities provide opportunities for children's development in the cognitive, physical, emotional and social domains. As a preschool teacher, you will want to consider each child's interests and abilities as you choose activities to include in the lessons.

The illustrations in this curriculum should be used as visual aids, not as coloring pages. Think about ways to use the illustrations as posters or picture cards. Learning theory suggests that preschoolers are not ready to color black-line pictures.

The activities in this curriculum are designed to teach the importance of respect and consideration for all people, regardless of gender or ethnic or religious background. As a preschool teacher, you will want to offer children of both sexes the opportunity to participate in a variety of activities.

Suggested books, songs, poems, rhymes and fingerplays were selected with a concern to avoid ethnic and gender stereotyping. Religious books, songs and poems were not included out of respect for religious diversity. The activities and lists were also developed with an awareness that there are many kinds of families.

Literature on early childhood education has recently reflected concern about the violence children are exposed to through war toys and the media. The activities and lists provided in this curriculum encourage peace education, with a belief that peace education contributes to individual health.

Ideally, young children should not have to protect themselves from substance abuse. Young children should not have to decide what to do if they find a weapon. Young children should not have to experience violence in their homes. But some do. Adults have a responsibility to provide a safe and secure world for children, but unfortunately, some adults do not fulfill this responsibility. Recognizing that young children are often confronted with these and other unfair situations, this curriculum includes objectives that address such situations.

Some objectives are more complex than others. It has been a challenge to include developmentally appropriate activities. The activities presented address the problems children may encounter, while considering children's ability to comprehend the problems. For example: The substance abuse activities focus on helping children understand that too much of anything is not healthy.

Great care was taken to avoid activities that may frighten or confuse young children. The preschool teacher is encouraged to be sensitive to and respectful of individual and community values in implementing the curriculum.

Providing preschool children with experiences that reinforce the role they play in caring for their health is an important task. Such experiences will add to children's understanding and appreciation of good health. This curriculum is designed for preschool teachers seeking both the means and materials to address this important educational topic.

Learning Strategies

Young children are comfortable with routine. They feel secure and gain confidence when participating in songs, games or activities that are familiar to them. Children also thrive on activities that extend their learning and stimulate thinking. A good mixture of activities for young children includes an established routine plus a few surprises in the form of new activities.

The learning strategies described here are common in many early childhood programs. These descriptions provide background and basic information about how to do specific activities, such as make a collage.

For each objective in this curriculum, suggestions are provided for ways to use these strategies to enhance children's learning. Each objective also includes new ideas for additional learning experiences.

Brainstorming

Brainstorming helps children develop thinking and creative skills. It involves listing all ideas a group or individual may have regarding a topic. The rules are simple:

- List *every* idea, no matter what it is.

- Don't judge any of the ideas.

- Don't discuss any of the ideas during the brainstorming.

- It's okay to repeat an idea or to say something similar.

Start the activity by explaining what brainstorming is. Tell children to think of as many ideas as they can.

Then write down all the ideas the children offer. Keep asking children for more ideas during the activity. When the list is finished, read the list. Point to each item as you read it.

Circle Share

During circle share, children are invited to talk one at a time about the suggested topic. Every child should have the opportunity to share. If this makes the activity too long for the children, adapt circle share one of the following ways:

- Have some children share at one circle time and others later that day. Be sure children who don't get a turn know that they will later, and when.

- Have small groups of different children meet at the same or different times.

Select children randomly to share rather than going in order from left to right. When children are aware of the order, they often pay more attention to that than to listening.

At the beginning of circle share, remind children that everyone will get a turn if they want one. Remind them that everyone is to listen while each person has a turn. You should model listening. Allow children time to think about their ideas before speaking.

Children learn to speak in front of others, use language, express themselves and listen through the circle share activity. They also learn new information.

Classroom Guests

Classroom guests are one way to share information with children. This method can also involve families and the community. Consider the following points when selecting classroom guests.

First, the purpose of the guest or the visit must be decided ahead of time. When you've determined the purpose, such as preparing for dental screening, look for someone who can serve that purpose. Is this person knowledgeable on the topic and interested in children?

When selecting visitors, consider gender, cultural backgrounds, ages, etc. Invite a diverse group of guests. When you contact possible guests, explain your need and the children's interest and abilities and suggest times for the visit.

When you find the appropriate guest, schedule and confirm the visit. You may want to meet with the guest to help plan the activity. Encourage guests to bring props and to dress in costumes or uniforms relating to their topics.

Prepare children for the visit. Explain the purpose of the visit. Remind children to listen and to be polite. Allow children to help decide what you and they can do to make the visitor feel welcome. Take a picture of each guest, so you can use the picture to extend the learning process after the visit.

After the visit, provide time for the children to react. This reaction time will be more valuable if you have prepared questions for the children to answer. For example: If the visitor is a dental assistant, ask questions such as: Have you ever been to a dentist? Do you brush your teeth at home? Why is it important to brush your teeth?

Follow-up activities can help you evaluate the usefulness of the experience. A thank-you note from you as well as from the class is a good way to show your appreciation.

Use your imagination and knowledge of your children and your resources in deciding which guests would be appropriate and when. Classroom guests expose children to information and ideas beyond the classroom. Guests also give children the opportunity to have first-hand experiences with a variety of people.

Collages

A collage is a picture made by pasting or gluing materials to a surface. Materials can include torn or cut paper, cloth, found objects, pictures from magazines or many other things. Either you or the children can determine the colors, shapes and sizes of the materials.

Provide different background surfaces, such as plywood, construction paper, poster board, oak tag, wallpaper samples, etc. Children can make individual collages, or the group can make a large one.

This curriculum contains many suggested themes for collages. Use your imagination and knowledge and your available supplies to decide on collage activities. Consider changing the collage materials each time the activity is used.

Children develop organization and classification skills through making collages. Fine motor skills are further enhanced by cutting, tearing and gluing. Group collages will also give children the opportunity to work as a team.

Collections

Collections offer children the opportunity to gather information and assemble it. Many items—such as rocks, blue things, shiny things, or pictures of flowers—can be collected.

Making collections encourages children to learn categorization of size, color, shape and other characteristics. Before children begin a collection, they must be able to discriminate between objects that fit into the collection and those that do not.

Collections can be kept in a variety of ways, depending on the type of collection. Collections can be kept in notebooks, shoe boxes, egg cartons, shadow boxes, etc.

A collection can be a class project or an individual one. If it's a class project, make it clear from the beginning what will happen to the items collected when the collection is finished.

If the items are to be returned to the finder or owner, be sure children register their items with you. You will need a system for keeping track of who brought what items. One method is to take a picture of each item. Another solution is to explain that all contributions will become property of the class.

Cooking with Children

Children learn many things from cooking experiences. They hear new words such as *grate;* they observe changes in food as it is cooked, stirred or frozen; they read recipes; they learn about measurement; and they taste nutritious foods.

Prior to the cooking experience, select a recipe. Write the recipe on a large piece of paper and illustrate it. Be sure to avoid foods that may cause allergic reactions in any of the children. Purchase food and gather your implements (blender, grater, peeler, bowls, cups, etc.).

The first cooking experience should be simple and include only a few ingredients and perhaps no heat. The children should do almost all of the cooking with the teacher providing guidance.

After a few sessions, no-heat cooking can become a learning center activity for children to do alone. Use pictures or a tape player to guide children through the experience. Remember that children should always wash their hands before touching food or utensils.

Discovery Box

A discovery box is any decorated, closed box with a hole large enough for a child to put one hand into easily. There may even be two or more holes—so a child can put in both hands or two children can put their hands in at the same time.

Either you or the children may decorate the box. Decorations should be bright and cheerful, so children will not be afraid to put their hands in the box. The box can be redecorated to keep the children's interest.

The discovery box can be used with both large or small groups with direct supervision, or it may be placed in a learning center. Place a variety of objects relating to the selected topic inside the box. Introduce the discovery box activity to create curiosity. After the children reach into the box, encourage discussion about the object.

Use your imagination, knowledge of your children and available resource materials when selecting objects for discovery box activities. The discovery box stimulates children's thinking and imagination, develops fine motor skills and encourages language development.

Field Trips

A field trip can provide an enjoyable opportunity for children to learn first hand. It can also be a way of involving the children's families and the community. This experience, if selected and planned well, can be one of the most worthwhile activities provided for children.

A major consideration when deciding on a field trip is the purpose. Is the purpose to introduce a topic, make a point or reach closure on a unit?

When the purpose has been decided, other considerations determine whether a trip is the best method for fulfilling the purpose. Would all the children benefit from the trip? Is there an appropriate place to visit that would welcome your class? How long has it been since your children were on a field trip?

If your answers to these questions indicate the need for a trip, check with your supervisor about obtaining permission or information. Next, contact possible places and people to visit. Explain the purpose of the visit and the children's interests and abilities. Suggest possible times for visiting.

When you find the trip that is most appropriate, schedule and confirm a time and date. Now you are ready to plan ways to prepare children, inform parents, arrange transportation, etc.

Tell the children about the trip and the reason for it. Let them help you plan and get ready for it. Children can help by taking the permission note home for approval.

The note should explain the trip and its purpose, invite family members to attend and state any special arrangements. Ask parents or guardians to complete the attached permission form and return it by the specified date. Your program may have its own procedures regarding permission forms.

Arrange for transportation. Be prepared for emergencies. Have enough adults, and take emergency phone numbers and emergency cards for the children. Before leaving, establish with the children and other adults the rules and responsibilities for everyone. Use travel time wisely, so the trip is an enjoyable learning experience.

After returning to the classroom, provide time for the children to react to the trip. Follow-up activities can help you evaluate the trip. A thank-you note from the teachers as well as one from the class is a good way to let the host or hostess know he or she is appreciated. Thank-you notes should also be written to parents and volunteers.

This curriculum includes several suggestions for trips. Use your imagination and knowledge of your children and your community to decide on appropriate field trips.

Language Experience Story

Children create language experience stories based on their experience. Provide an idea or prop to help children get started. If the children have never written (told) stories, you may need to start with a sentence.

Write the child's story word-for-word as it is dictated. Do *not* correct the child or change the story. Say the letters and words as they are written.

The letters should be printed clearly using correct manuscript (letter) form. Read each sentence as it is finished. Read the entire story whenever the child asks and when the story is over.

After the story is written, the child may want to illustrate it. Another variation is to draw a picture first and then have the child develop a story about the picture. Stories can also be told on a tape player for variety.

Language experience stories encourage children to express themselves and to develop creativity and improve their use of language. Writing children's stories for them is an appropriate reading readiness activity.

Lotto

Lotto is a game in which children match cards on a game board. Many different pictures or colors can appear on the cards. Although lotto games are sold commercially, they are very simple to make. The steps to make a lotto game are as follows:

- Mark off six (or any number) equal sections on two large sheets of heavy paper.

- On one sheet, draw or paste six different pictures. This is your game board.

- Draw or paste the same pictures on the second sheet and cut the sections apart to make six (or more) cards.

- Cover the game board and each card with clear contact paper to make it more durable.

Children will probably experiment and play with the game before they begin to match the cards to the game board. The game can be played with direct supervision in a large or small group before being added to a learning center.

Children develop matching skills by playing lotto, and learn about game playing. They also develop fine motor skills by manipulating the game cards.

Make a Puzzle

Have children draw, trace or cut pictures from magazines to paste on heavy pieces of paper. Cover the pictures with clear contact paper or laminate them to make them more durable. Cut the paper into several pieces of various shapes (not just squares). On another sheet of heavy paper, or on the inside of a manila folder, put each picture back together.

The next step is to create an outline of each piece, so children can work the puzzle by themselves. First, draw an outline of the entire picture. Next, remove one piece at a time and draw lines around the opening. Staple an envelope to the back of the folder or cardboard to store the pieces in.

Children may need help cutting puzzle pieces, or they will sometimes cut their pictures into too many small pieces. Assist children who are unable to use scissors safely.

Use your imagination, knowledge of your children and available resources to choose ideas for puzzles. Children develop fine motor skills in making puzzles. They also develop pride in producing a toy they can use over and over.

Mobiles

A mobile is a hanging object with parts that are set in motion by air currents. There are many kinds of mobiles. The kind you choose to make should depend on the skills and concepts being taught, the children's interests and available materials. Mobiles can be made by hanging pictures or objects from a stick or tree branch, a coat hanger, a paper plate or a pie tin.

Suggestions regarding topics for mobiles are made throughout this curriculum. However, the selection of materials for mobiles is limited only by your imagination and common sense. The size of the objects should be too large for children to swallow, and objects should not be poisonous.

Children learn to categorize items, develop fine motor skills and use their creativity when working on a mobile.

Paper People

Paper people are large paper dolls that represent the children. Provide a large sheet of butcher paper or newsprint for each child. Have each child lie down on the paper, leaving a few inches of paper at the top. The teacher, a parent or another child should draw the outline of the child. Display all the paper people.

This curriculum includes several paper people activities. You may want to store the paper people or let the children make additional paper people for different activities.

Paper people help children build a positive self-image. They can also be used to reinforce the specific curriculum content.

Problem Solving

Both adults and children experience ongoing situations that require problem solving. Children develop cognitive skills by seeking solutions to concrete problems. Teaching children problem-solving skills will decrease discipline problems, as children learn to solve problems peacefully and independently.

To learn problem solving, children need to see you model it and encourage it everyday in the classroom. You will need to help children learn how to identify the problem, generate ideas, evaluate the ideas and make a decision.

Begin the problem-solving activities by describing a situation and asking children what they could do. You might also ask what would happen if they did that. Keep asking questions to give children practice at seeing possible consequences.

Roleplay

In a roleplay situation, children try out roles of other persons or try their own roles in various situations. They should have freedom to act out their own way, without memorizing lines, etc.

Try to help children understand that roleplaying is make-believe. Remember that to young children, play is real. It may be easier to introduce roleplaying by giving children a topic or situation and saying, "Show us what you would do if..." or "Show us something that...."

Young children have difficulty seeing situations from another person's perspective. Therefore, it is important to provide each child with the opportunity to reverse roles when roleplaying involves more than one person.

Roleplaying is useful and helps children express themselves. However, it is far more important for you to help children deal with real situations and feelings that occur naturally.

Someone Says

Someone Says is similar to the traditional Simon Says game, except the leader uses his or her own name and the children are never out. For example: "Kevin says, 'Stretch your arms out.'" The children are not supposed to follow the command unless "Kevin says."

In Simon Says, children are out if they make a mistake. But in this version, children are not out. When a child makes a mistake, *everyone* turns around once and then is ready for the next command.

Someone Says allows children to use their own names, which builds self-esteem. Someone Says also gives children practice in listening to and following directions. Since there are no losers, everyone benefits throughout the game.

Spinning Wheel

Cut a cardboard circle approximately ten inches in diameter. Divide it into five equal parts. Draw or glue a picture relating to the topic on each of the sections. Cover the circle with clear contact paper or laminate it to make it more durable.

Punch a small hole in the center of the circle. Make an arrow with a hole punched in the center. Match the hole on the arrow and the circle and connect with a paper fastener. Check to see that the arrow spins when you flip it. If it doesn't, you may have fastened it too tightly.

To start the game, spin the arrow and see what picture it lands on. Have children tell you about the picture. Children can also toss a bean bag, hop or do some other activity after they tell you about a picture.

If the topic has right and wrong answers, the back of the card can give a code for answers. Use colors or smile pictures to show correct answers. (If you are aware of any child with color blindness, do not use colors for the code.)

Surveys

Surveys provide children with the opportunity to gather and organize information. Surveys also encourage children to categorize their findings. They make children aware of differences and similarities.

Surveys can be active experiments on various subjects. It is important to let children seek answers and learn by their own experience instead of just being told something.

Chart the results of each survey. Use a different type of chart each time. For example, use bar graphs and a list of the results. Discuss the findings as a class.

Surveys are recommended throughout this curriculum. Explain the purpose of the survey to the children and assist them in processing the information they gather.

If the survey extends beyond your classroom, you may want to inform those who will be surveyed and make necessary arrangements. If others understand the reason for the survey, they may be more likely to help children gather information without feeling that you or the children are being nosy.

Walks

A short walk on or near the school grounds can be an enjoyable and valuable learning experience for children. Taking a walk requires little planning, but it will be a more beneficial experience if some planning occurs. Prepare children by explaining the purpose of the trip. Occasionally, let children help you plan for that purpose.

Before the first walk, discuss the safety rules to be followed (such as walk, stay behind the teacher, etc.). Children can help you make the rules and discuss reasons for rules. Always review these rules before taking a walk.

We recommend that you obtain written permission from parents or guardians if you travel off the school property. Walking on a part of the playground that is not used daily is special to young children, so you may choose to stay on school property. Then you wouldn't need written permission.

Take a camera on the walk and take pictures related to the purpose of the walk. Use the pictures in the classroom to remind children about the walk.

After the walk, provide opportunities for children to discuss and share the experience by drawing, dictating stories or roleplaying. The curriculum includes specific suggestions for walks, but be creative and develop additional ideas.

Walks provide the opportunity for exercise and fresh air. They also give children the opportunity to learn from the surrounding environment and develop knowledge related to the purpose of the walk.

Where Does It Go?

Where Does It Go? is a classification game in which children sort objects or pictures according to specified characteristics. The number of groups depends on the topic and the abilities of the children.

The objects or pictures are placed in designated areas such as boxes, trays, baskets or a circle made of yarn, tape or paper. An example of grouping would be all red things in one basket and all blue things in another.

This game can be played with teacher direction in small groups as well as with individual children. It can also be available for children to experiment with during learning center times.

Using the game first in a group is a good way to show how it works. Objects and pictures for grouping should be changed regularly in order to keep the children's interest.

This curriculum includes many suggestions for objects and pictures to use in this activity. Use your imagination and your knowledge of your children and available materials to decide on the details of the game.

Children develop thinking and sorting skills through playing Where Does It Go?

Learning Centers

Learning centers are areas that are arranged to encourage children to actively explore materials and interact with others. They can be inside or outside the classroom. They are a significant part of any preschool classroom.

Learning centers should be carefully planned to ensure that a developmentally appropriate environment is provided for young children. How materials are displayed and labeled is important. You can facilitate children's learning in the learning centers by interacting with the children, asking open-ended questions, making suggestions, assisting children and guiding them in their activities.

You should schedule classes to include time for children to use the learning centers every day. The amount of time allotted will depend on the number of hours each classroom is open. A large proportion of the day should be scheduled for learning center time.

Any learning center that stays in the classroom or outside on an ongoing basis is referred to in this curriculum as a Traditional Learning Center. The traditional centers are: art, blocks, housekeeping, manipulative and science. (Manipulative is sometimes called fine motor, or it may be limited to puzzles.) Each objective in this curriculum includes suggestions for materials to add to traditional learning centers.

Many suggestions are made for the five traditional centers listed above. If your learning centers are different from those listed, determine which of your centers is the best place for each suggestion. Select those that you and your children will enjoy most.

In addition to these centers, you can gather or make materials to create new Special Learning Centers. Specific guidance and examples are suggested in this curriculum. Of course, you are encouraged to use your own imagination and knowledge of available resources as well.

Special learning centers provide children the opportunity to learn new concepts and look at old ones in a new way. They reinforce concepts that you are teaching in other ways. Special learning centers will keep children interested in exploring and learning.

Although books are used as a traditional learning center in most classrooms, they are not included in these learning center recommendations because a separate book list is provided. We recommend that resource books be added for each unit.

Many of the activities in the curriculum can be included in the learning centers. Be creative, and make your learning centers a pleasurable learning experience for your children.

Suggested Teaching Sequence

A teaching sequence is intended to provide assistance to preschool teachers. It should not be seen as limiting teachers' freedom to schedule the learning objectives based on the needs of the children in their classrooms and their program goals.

Since many preschools operate on a nine-month schedule, a sequence including all objectives for this time period is presented. Because other preschools are open year-round, the learning activities most appropriate for repeating and/or extending are outlined in a separate sequence.

Geographic location and relative timing of community activities may influence when specific learning objectives are best addressed. For example: The Head Start program encourages daily brushing of teeth by the children. Participants in this program may want to present the learning objective related to brushing teeth early in the school year. If your community has scheduled an event such as a Drug-Free Awareness Week or the Just Say No campaign, you may want to present the learning objectives on medicines and substance use prevention to coincide with community activities.

The suggested teaching sequence begins in September, when many preschool programs begin. Adjust your specific teaching sequence to fit your own nine- or twelve-month schedule.

Here We Go...Watch Me Grow!

September

- What I Like About Myself — Objective 4
- Growing My Way — Objective 2
- Social Behavior — Objective 6

October

- Safety Rules — Objective 23
- Caring for the Environment — Objective 34
- Helping at Home — Objective 11
- Family Jobs — Objective 13

November

- Jobs and Careers — Objective 14
- Health Helpers — Objective 33
- Feeling Sad — Objective 5
- Body Parts and the Senses — Objective 1

December

- What to Put in Your Mouth — Objective 24
- Sharing Food and Drinks — Objective 20
- The Basic Four Food Groups — Objective 16

January

- Nutritious Snacks — Objective 15
- Family Members — Objective 12
- What Are Commercials? — Objective 28
- Using Car Seats and Seat Belts — Objective 26

February

- What to Wear — Objective 9
- Cover Your Mouth and Nose — Objective 18
- Exercise Helps Us Grow — Objective 10
- Brush Your Teeth — Objective 8

March

- Wash Your Hands — Objective 17
- Identifying Emotions — Objective 3
- When You're Hurt — Objective 7
- Medicines That Prevent Disease — Objective 19

April

- When to Take Medicine — Objective 29
- Who Should Give Medicine — Objective 30
- Tobacco's Harmful Effects — Objective 31
- Substance Use Prevention — Objective 32

Here We Go...Watch Me Grow!

May

- Community Safety Helpers — Objective 22
- Never Play with Weapons — Objective 25
- In Case of Fire — Objective 27
- Traffic Signs and Signals — Objective 21

June

- What I Like About Myself — Objective 4
- Growing My Way — Objective 2
- Social Behavior — Objective 6
- Safety Rules — Objective 23

July

- Caring for the Environment — Objective 34
- What to Put in Your Mouth — Objective 24
- Nutritious Snacks — Objective 15
- Family Members — Objective 12

August

- Using Car Seats and Seat Belts — Objective 26
- Wash Your Hands — Objective 17
- Identifying Emotions — Objective 3
- When You're Hurt — Objective 7

1.

Growth and Development

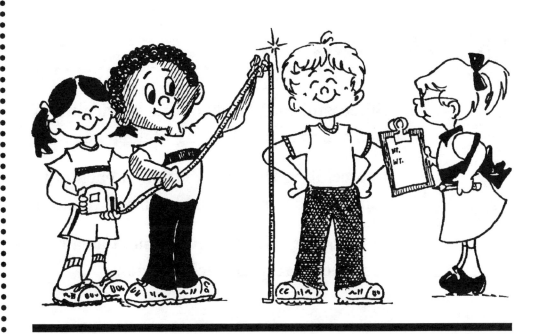

Growth and Development

This unit will help children understand growth and development and how the two are related. As their bodies grow, children begin to develop new abilities and skills. Their behavior and the choices they make can help their bodies grow and develop properly.

This unit introduces children to the structure and function of body systems. For example: The respiratory system controls breathing; the digestive system deals with eating; and the circulatory system pumps blood to the body. Each system needs the other systems, and each contributes to the overall healthy functioning of the body.

Lifestyle Goals

Successful completion of this curriculum will put children on the road to achieving lifelong goals of:

- appreciating the contribution of each of the body systems to the survival and health of the total system;

- viewing growth and development as a lifelong process fostered by responsible behavior.

Here We Go...Watch Me Grow!

Objective 1
Body Parts
and the Senses

Children will be able to identify one body part primarily associated with each of the five senses.

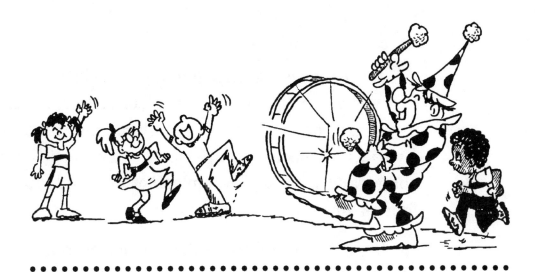

The purpose of this objective is to help children realize the importance of the five senses: taste, touch, sight, smell and hearing. The senses are used for recognition and communication. Each sense organ (skin/finger, eye, nose, tongue, ear) can act independently. The senses also work together. For example: If food *looks* good and *smells* good, we will want to *taste* it.

Discuss the need we have for our senses and how we compensate if we do not have use of a sense. Explain that some people do not have the use of one or more senses for a variety of reasons. Explain that there are times when we lose use of a sense temporarily, for example, when the lights are out.

Since the senses work together, they can even compensate for each other when one sense is lost.

Activities ....

Discovery Box

Touch: Ask children to put their hands in the Discovery Box and describe how an object feels. After describing the object and guessing what it is, children may take it out. Use a variety of objects that are hard or soft and different sizes, shapes and textures. Examples: cotton, sandpaper, sponge, fabrics, toys from the classroom.

Sight: Have children select an object from the box and place it on top of the Discovery Box. Children describe the objects according to what they see. Use objects of various colors, shapes, sizes, etc. Use both familiar and unfamiliar objects.

Smell: Have children close their eyes and select an object from the Discovery Box. Children then describe the smell and guess what the object is. Examples: perfume on a tissue, garlic clove, cinnamon stick, peppermint candy.

Taste: Have children close their eyes and select an object from the Discovery Box to taste. Children then describe the taste and guess what the object is. After they guess, children may look at the object. Use foods that are sweet, sour, salty, etc., such as raw fruits or vegetables, breads, pretzels.

Place only one food at a time in the box on a paper plate. To reduce waiting, this should be an individual or small group activity. Remember to have children wash their hands before playing the game.

Hearing: Have children put their hands in the box and cause the object to make a noise (such as by shaking, squeezing or flattening it). Ask children to describe the sound and guess what the object is. After they guess, children may look at the object.

Objects to use include items in a small container for children to shake, baby rattle, crackly (cellophane) paper or a pet squeak toy. Some items, such as a whistle, may not make a sound in the box, but can be taken out to make noise.

Walks

Touch: Take along a container for each child to collect things that can be touched during the walk. Talk with children about respecting living things and other people's property. For example: It is not appropriate for children to pick flowers from the neighbor's garden unless they have permission. Be certain that children do not pick up sharp objects (such as glass) or cigarette butts.

Sight: Go for a walk and encourage children to look above and below them to see things they might not have noticed before. Take binoculars and/or magnifying glasses to use during the walk.

Smell: Encourage children to smell different scents during a walk. Suggest that they try smelling things up close, such as trees, flowers, etc. Watch out for bees!

Taste: Prepare a tasty snack, and go on a walk to a nearby picnic area that is safe and attractive. Talk about taste. Does food taste different when eaten outside?

Hearing: Take a listening walk. Encourage children to listen to sounds made by animals, people, machines, etc. Take a stethoscope and listen to a tree, the ground and other things.

Paper People

Touch: Discuss with children the parts of the body that they use to feel things. Children can outline the paper people hands with a darker or brighter color crayon, or they can just trace the paper hands with their own fingers. Help children understand that they feel with *all* their skin, not just their fingers.

Sight: Discuss with children the parts of the body that they use to see things. Children can draw eyes on the paper people.

Smell: Discuss with children the part of the body that they use to smell things. Children can draw noses on the paper people.

Taste: Discuss with children the part of the body that they use to taste things. Children can draw mouths on the paper people. Talk about how the tongue is behind the lips (inside the mouth).

Hearing: Discuss with children the parts of the body that they use to hear sounds. Children can draw ears on the paper people.

Collages

Touch: Use things collected on a Sense of Touch Walk or other objects to make a collage of things to feel.

Sight: Make a collage with pictures of eyes cut from magazines. Use a large piece of paper cut in the shape of an eye for the background sheet.

Smell: Make a group collage of smells, using pictures from magazines or items having a fragrance, such as peppermint candies, scented facial tissues or cotton balls sprayed with perfume.

Taste: Make individual collages using magazine pictures of tastes the children like and dislike. Fold the background paper in half and paste the likes on one side and the dislikes on the other side.

Hearing: Make a collage of things children can hear, using pictures of records, radios, cars, etc. Use a large piece of paper cut in the shape of an ear for the background sheet.

Touch and Tell

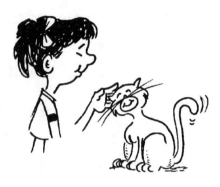

Have children sit in a circle with their hands behind their backs. Pass around an object. After the object has been all the way around the circle, ask each child to describe it and try to guess what it is. Use different objects such as a feather, a rock, a cotton ball, etc.

I See Something

One child says, "I see something and it's *(describe it, such as color or shape)*." Other children try to guess what it is. The game can be made easier by limiting the objects to be described to four or five designated ones or by limiting the "see something" area to a corner or wall or other small area of the room.

Children must tell you what they are describing, so they can't change their minds when someone guesses the object. The child who guesses correctly does not become the next child to describe an object. All children should have a turn describing objects, whether they guess correctly or not, so the teacher should choose the next leader.

Smell and Tell

Provide small containers of substances with familiar and distinctive odors (perfume, peppermint, etc.). Let children smell each container and tell what they think it is. An alternative is to have more than one container of each smell, and let children match the smells.

Use unbreakable containers that cannot be seen through. Punch holes in the lids so children can smell the contents. If using spices or powder, you can place a small circle of nylon stocking over the container opening to prevent spills.

Taste Time

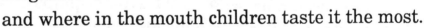

Let children look in a mirror to see their taste buds. Provide different foods for children to apply to the tip, middle, side and back of their tongues. Discuss how the food tastes and where in the mouth children taste it the most.

Provide water to drink between each tasting. Foods to taste include sugar, lemon juice, vinegar, nutmeg, bitter chocolate, etc. Consider any food allergies children may have when selecting foods.

Shake and Listen

Provide small colored containers to make shakers. Fill each one with substances such as salt, macaroni, rice, pinto beans, etc. Use one substance per shaker and two shakers for each substance. Let children shake one container and describe the sound. Then they can find the other shaker with the same sound.

A Touching Experience

Tell children to touch one body part with another body part. Examples: Touch your ears with your hands; touch your toe with your fingers; touch your knees with your elbows.

Toe-Paint

Toe-paint just as you would finger-paint. Use powdered tempera for color, and add salt or rice for texture. Explain that we can feel with many parts of our bodies, but we use our hands a lot when we touch. This activity shows children they can use their feet to touch. Talk about how the paint feels on their feet as children paint.

Goggles

Ask children to put on goggles that have been lightly sprayed with paint. (Be considerate of children's fears, and do not insist that they wear the goggles.) Then hold up pictures for children to identify. An alternative is to turn out the lights and ask children what they can see. Discuss how it feels to be unable to see clearly.

Tastes

Ask children to hold their noses and taste different foods. Discuss whether the food tasted different. Taste a raw potato, then taste a raw potato with salt. Point out that we have some control over flavoring foods. However, note that some people cannot taste any flavors.

Earplugs

Have children wear earphones or earplugs or hold their hands over their ears while they listen to directions you give. Discuss how it feels to be unable to hear clearly.

Field Trips

Visit an optician's office. Point out that there are many different types of glasses to help people see more clearly.

Visit an audiologist's office or hearing aid office. Explain that there are some ways to help people hear more clearly.

Traditional Learning Centers

Art

Add sandpaper to draw or paint on, chalk to draw with, a tray of salt or cornmeal to draw in and play dough for creating. Mix different colors of food coloring with glue and place a container of each in the art center. Add containers of feathers and scraps of different materials such as felt, lace and ribbon for children to use in making collages. Add sand mixed with different colors of tempera, and coffee grounds for texture collages.

Blocks

Add beans or small rocks for hauling in trucks. Add vehicles that make noise, such as firetrucks, police cars, tractors, etc.

Housekeeping

Add candles, a lantern, flashlights and eyeglasses without lenses. Add flowers for the table, powder for the dolls, clothes sprayed with perfume or after-shave cologne. Add potatoes and carrots and a potato peeler. Add a transistor radio, an alarm clock and an eggbeater. Add large clip-on earrings to encourage discussions about ears.

Manipulative

Add puzzles relating to each sense.

Science

Add magnifying glasses, a box with a small hole in it to look through, flashlights of various types, binoculars and a telescope. Add a tape player with blank tapes for children to record on and/or tapes of sounds children can listen to and identify. Encourage a variety of guesses—the right answer is not important. Add a large seashell and bells or other instruments.

Add a water table, sand table, rice table or bean table. If tables are not available, use buckets, dishpans or other containers.

Resources

• •

More information on these resources can be found starting on p. 261.

Books

Sight

Brown Bear, Brown Bear,
   What Do You See?
Eye Book
It Looked Like Spilt Milk
What Spot?

Hearing

The Ear Book
I Know an Old Lady
It's Too Noisy
Too Much Noise

Smell

Moon Man

Taste

Blueberries for Sal
Bread and Jam for Frances
The Carrot Seed

Touch

Pat the Bunny

All Senses

First Delights
A Hole Is to Dig
My Five Senses

Songs

Sight

All of Us Will Shine
   Flowers
Circle Around
   The Monster Song
Learning Basic Skills
   Stop, Look and Listen
One Light, One Sun
   De Colores
   Walk Outside
Singable Songs
   Down by the Bay
Sing Your Sillies Out
   All the Colors of the Rainbow

Hearing

Everything Grows
   Let's Make Some Noise
Hug the Earth
   Tickle Train
Learning Basic Skills
   Stop, Look and Listen
One Light, One Sun
   Down on Grandpa's Farm
   Time to Sing
Peace Is the World Smiling
   Voices
Singable Songs
   Old McDonald Had a Band

Here We Go...Watch Me Grow!

Teaching Peace
   Listen

Smell
All of Us Will Shine
   Flowers
Hug the Earth
   Garbage Blues
When My Shoes Are Loose
   Open Flower

Taste
One Light, One Sun
   Apples and Bananas

Touch
Everything Grows
   Bathtime
   Teddy Bear Hug

Hug the Earth
   Skin

All Senses
All of Us Will Shine
   My Body Belongs to Me
Circle Around
   Bear Hunt
Hug the Earth
   Hug the Earth
One Light, One Sun
   One Light, One Sun
Voyage for Dreamers
   Walk in Beauty

Poems, Rhymes and Fingerplays

Sight
Finger Frolics
   Sight
   Stars
Where the Sidewalk Ends
   It's Dark in Here

Hearing
Finger Frolics
   My Fingers
   Ready to Listen
   The Wind

Smell
Finger Frolics
   My Mother's Bouquet

Where the Sidewalk Ends
   Sarah Cynthia Sylvia Stout
     Would Not Take the
     Garbage Out

Taste
Finger Frolics
   The Four Food Groups

Touch
Finger Frolics
   Head and Shoulder
   Ten Little Fingers
   Warm Hands
   The Wind

All Senses

Finger Frolics
  Hand on Myself
  How Many

Where the Sidewalk Ends
  The Loser

Objective 2
Growing My Way

Children will be able to explain that every child grows and develops in his or her own way.

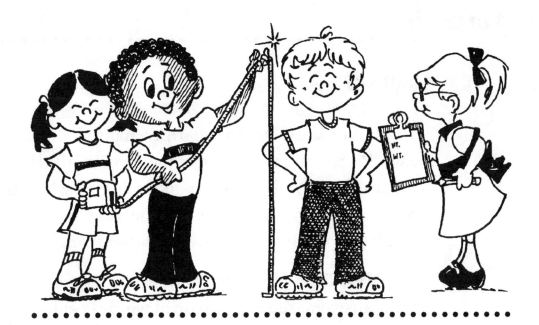

The purpose of this objective is to help children identify and accept similarities and differences among people. The basic makeup of everyone's body is the same. Everybody needs to eat, sleep and breathe. However, growth rate and individual abilities vary for many reasons.

Everyone has strengths of some kind, but no one excels at everything. For example: A child may be able to run very fast, but may not be able to jump rope well. Children have individual interests, and they are usually best at activities they enjoy.

Some growth and developmental differences are related to disabling conditions. Children with such conditions can develop other strengths. For example: A child with cerebral palsy may have difficulty with motor activities such as running, but may be able to climb well. The same child may excel in reading and solving puzzles.

Activities

Surveys

Survey the children regarding likes, dislikes and interests. Prepare a large piece of paper with all the children's names on it. Ask children individually what they like, dislike and are interested in. You may need to give the children specific possibilities to select from for the survey.

Draw little pictures by children's names to represent their answers. You can also print words beside the pictures.

After you survey all the children, talk about likenesses and differences in the group. Ask children if they can remember what they used to like or dislike or were interested in. Have there been any changes? Why or why not?

Body Prints

Make a print of each child's thumb, finger, hand, toe or foot. Press the body part onto a washable ink or paint pad and then onto paper. Display the prints and have children look for similarities and differences. Explain that everyone's print is his or her own and no one else has one exactly like it.

Make more than one print of the same body part and let children match their prints. To simplify this process, have only a few prints from which to choose. Write names on the back or front of the paper to make it easier.

Which Ones?

This game starts with everyone sitting down. Then ask, for example, "Who likes ice cream?" Tell the children who like ice cream to stand up and then sit down. Use likes and dislikes that will show similarities and differences.

Can You?

You need to be aware of activities that each child can do well, so that this is a positive game. Ask children questions such as, "Can you run to that tree and back three times?" Have the children who think they can, do it. Use a variety of activities that all children are good at. This game can be played with teams as well as with individuals.

Paper People

Measure each child's height. Write the height on the paper person near the head. Draw a line beside the outline from the feet to the head to show how height is measured. At the middle and the end of the school year, measure children again and compare the growth. You may also want to record weight at these times.

Discuss growth and physical likenesses and differences of the children. Children can be sensitive to differences in height, weight and other physical characteristics, so be cautious in your discussion.

Someone Says

Give tasks that will be easy for everyone, hard for everyone and in-between tasks. Discuss how some things are easy for some of us and hard for others. Examples (difficulty may depend on age of children): stand on one foot, jump up and down, turn around, whistle, etc.

Roleplay

Say to each child, "Show us something that is easy for you to do."

Circle Share

Let children tell about something that is difficult for them to do. Explain that some things can be learned, but sometimes we aren't able to learn certain things. For example: A blind person cannot learn to see; a short person cannot learn to be tall.

Classroom Guests

Invite a parent or other family member to bring a baby to visit the class. Discuss the differences and likenesses among the baby and the children. Consider differences in physical characteristics, interests and abilities.

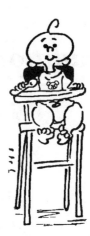

Special Learning Centers

Clothing and Shoe Store

Collect various clothes and shoes of different styles and sizes. Set up an area as a store. Provide a cash register and play money. You might also include scales, measuring tapes and a ruler for measuring for correct sizes. Encourage children to try on clothes that are too little and discuss how they have grown.

Bodybuilding

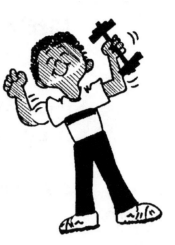

Set up an exercise center where children can strengthen their bodies by exercise. Add a mat to an area away from traffic. Post pictures of people exercising. Add exercise records and/or videotapes if appropriate.

Traditional Learning Centers

Art

Display famous art works, and encourage children to discuss the works they like or dislike. Pictures can be found in calendars, magazines, museum gift shops and catalogs.

Add new art materials, and encourage children to discuss what they like and dislike.

Add two kinds of clay or play dough, and ask children how the two kinds are alike and how they are different. Encourage children to feel, smell and look before responding.

Blocks

Add pictures of structures, and ask children which they like and dislike. Add new props of any kind, and encourage children to discuss what they like and dislike about the new things. Add props so there are two or more of each item. Talk about things that are alike.

Take pictures of the structures children build in the block center, and encourage the builders to talk about likenesses and differences.

Housekeeping

Add clothes of many styles for children to discuss. Add other props such as new rugs, pillows, tablecloths, etc., and encourage discussion. Ask children to compare the old items to the new ones. You may need to have the old items in sight for the comparisons.

Display pictures of people from different ethnic groups. Display pictures of people of various ages. Display pictures of people with disabling conditions. Encourage discussion.

Add dolls that could represent different ages and discuss the differences in growth.

Manipulative

Add puzzles that represent people from different ethnic groups and of different ages. If puzzles aren't available, make them from pictures and store in envelopes.

Add new manipulative toys, and encourage children to discuss how they are like the old ones. Examples include different beads or pegs.

Science

Add cups with water and provide food color for children to make colored water. Encourage discussion about likenesses and differences.

Provide seeds, soil and containers for planting seeds. Care for the plantings and watch them grow. Keep a chart of the watering and growth. Take pictures of the plants at different stages.

Resources

· ·

More information on these resources can be found starting on p. 261.

Books

Likenesses and Differences
Jo, Flo and Yolanda
People
The Twins Strike Back
The Ugly Duckling
You Are Special

Birth
How You Were Born
Wind Rose

Abilities
I Can, Can You?

Growing
The Carrot Seed
Daydreamers
Leo, the Late Bloomer
The Sheep Book
Why Am I Different?

Disabling Conditions
ABC-ing an Action Alphabet
Button in Her Ear
Grandma's Wheelchair
Like Me
My Favorite Place

Songs

Abilities

All of Us Will Shine
  All of Us Will Shine
  Everyone Is Differently Abled
  My Body Belongs to Me
Baby Beluga
  This Old Man
Everything Grows
  Ha Ha Thisaway
  Teddy Bear Hug
Voyage for Dreamers
  Many the Flowers
When My Shoes Are Loose
  Telephone
  When My Shoes Are Loose

Likenesses and Differences

Circle Around
  The Monster Song
Everything Grows
  Just Like the Sun
  Teddy Bear Hug
Hug the Earth
  Skin
One Light, One Sun
  Like Me and You
  One Light, One Sun
Peace Is the World Smiling
  Everybody is Somebody
  Kid's Peace Song
  Turn the World Around

Sing Your Sillies Out
  All the Colors of the Rainbow
Teaching Peace
  Hurray for the World
  Listen
  Places in the World
  Rapp Song
Travellin' with Ella Jenkins
  Greetings in Many Languages

Growing

All of Us Will Shine
  Flowers
Baby Beluga
  Oats and Beans and Barley
Everything Grows
  Everything Grows
Learning Basic Skills
  Posture Exercises
One Light, One Sun
  In My Garden
Singable Songs
  Wonder if I'm Growing?
Sing Your Sillies Out
  The Corn Song
When My Shoes Are Loose
  Every Year I Have a Birthday
  Open Flower
  Telephone

Poems, Rhymes and Fingerplays

Abilities

Finger Frolics
   If I Could Play
   My Arms
   Ten Little Fingers
   Things I Can Do
Where the Sidewalk Ends
   Jumping Rope
   Listen to the Mustn'ts
   Magic

Likes and Dislikes

Finger Frolics
   I Like To ...
Where the Sidewalk Ends
   Hector the Collector

Likenesses and Differences

Finger Frolics
   The Dinosaurs
   Very, Very Tall

Free to Be ... a Family
   The Little Boy and the Old
     Man
Where the Sidewalk Ends
   Colors
   Me and My Giant
   One Inch Tall

Growing

Finger Frolics
   Amphibians
   Growing Up
   Little Brown Seed
   Once There Was a Pumpkin
   Seeds

Disabling Conditions

Free to Be ... a Family
   The Biggest Problem (Is in
     Other People's Minds)
   Like Me
Where the Sidewalk Ends
   It's Dark in Here

2.

Mental and Emotional Health

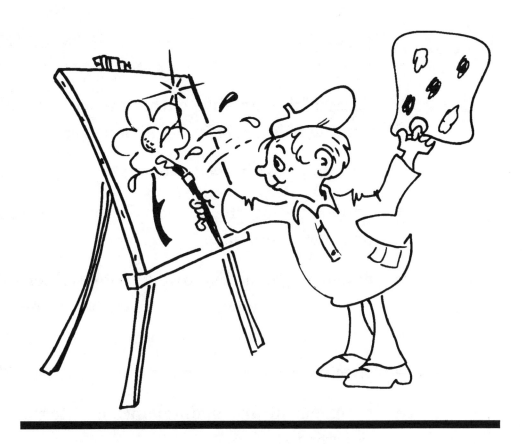

Mental and Emotional Health

Positive mental health includes the ability to apply problem-solving skills to the resolution of individual and family concerns. Children need to develop a positive self-concept and respect for the rights of others. Mental and emotional health also involve accepting responsibility for one's own health.

Lifestyle Goals

Successful completion of this curriculum will put children on the road to achieving lifelong goals of:

- attaining positive self-esteem;

- understanding the comfortable and appropriate expression of emotions;

- developing the ability to weigh potential benefits against possible consequences before choosing one action over another;

- effective communication and cooperation with others;

- development and maintenance of interpersonal relationships.

Here We Go...Watch Me Grow!

Objective 3
Identifying Emotions

Children will be able to identify the emotions of anger, happiness, sadness, excitement, love and fear.

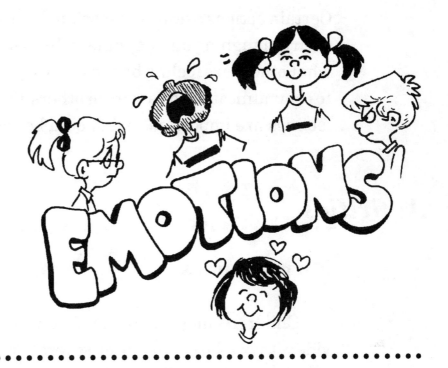

The purpose of this objective is to help children recognize that they may have different feelings in different situations. Two children in the same situation may feel differently.

All these different feelings are normal and healthy, within some boundaries of acceptability. For example: If Mieko breaks April's favorite toy, it is okay for April to feel mad or sad or even afraid that Mieko will break other toys. It is not okay for April to get so mad that she breaks Mieko's toys to get even.

Help children identify and accept their feelings of anger, happiness, sadness, excitement, love and fear. Discuss these emotions in the context of children's feelings for their families, friends and pets.

People may show their emotions through actions, such as crying when they are sad or smiling when they are happy. Certain actions are often associated with certain emotions, such as laughing and happiness. But we cannot always tell what others are feeling by the way they are acting. We need to communicate to be aware of others' feelings. Everybody's feelings are important and should be respected.

Activities
....

Mirror Games

Children enjoy looking at themselves in a mirror. Provide either a large mirror or several small mirrors for the children. Help children with the following activities.

Encourage children to practice making faces in a mirror. Suggest they make faces to show feeling happy, sad, angry, scared, excited, surprised, etc.

Make a face and let the children try to make a face like yours. Let them guess what emotion you are feeling to make your face look like that. Explain that they can only guess. They cannot be sure about your true feelings.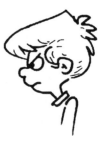

54

Have each child select and face a partner. One child makes a face; the other tries to make the same face. Children take turns making and copying faces to show emotions. You may need to help the children decide who will be first. You may also need to call out one emotion at a time and tell children when it is time to change turns.

Have children stand back to back with their partners while you call out an emotion. Both children make a face to match the emotion. They then turn to see each other's face and their own faces by looking in a mirror together.

Keep a picture beside a designated mirror. Children can make the face in the mirror that the picture makes them feel like. For example: A picture of a dog may make one child feel very happy, but it may remind another child of being scared. This picture can change often. Children can make the face at free time, on their way to someplace or one at a time as they leave the group to go to another activity.

Emotional Musical Chairs

To prepare for emotional musical chairs, line the chairs up as in traditional musical chairs, with enough chairs for all but one child. However, no more chairs are removed during the game.

Place pictures of faces showing different emotions in a box or basket. Have children move around the chairs as the music plays and try to find a seat when the music stops.

The child without a chair draws a picture out of the box and shows it to the other children. The child then tells what emotion he or she thinks the person in the picture is feeling. All the children then make faces and act out the emotion until the music starts again. Children move around the chairs again, and the game continues.

Structure the game so that no particular child is without a chair several times. Otherwise, he or she may be teased about being slow, or the other children may resent one child getting several turns to choose a picture.

One way to avoid this problem is to have enough chairs for everyone. When the music stops, you select the picture, or ask a different child to select a picture each time. If your group includes more than ten children, this could become a small group activity, or two groups can play at one time.

Mobiles

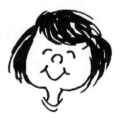

Let children make mobiles with things that make them happy. Pictures can be cut from magazines or objects can be collected.

Collages

Let children make collages of things that create a feeling of excitement. Pictures might include a circus, the ice cream truck, a new baby, thunderstorms, etc.

Surveys

Survey the children to see what makes them angry. Record each child's name and response.

Circle Share

Sadness: Ask children to tell about something that makes them sad. Explain that we all are sad sometimes and it is okay to feel sad.

Fear: Invite children to talk about something that they are afraid of. Explain that we all are afraid of some things. Discuss ways of overcoming fears.

Roleplays

Tell children to act out something they like.

Invite children to show the group something that makes them angry.

Ask each child to show how Kevin would act if something surprised him.

Ask each child to show how Mieko would feel at a party where there were presents for her.

Ask each child to show how April would feel if Kevin sneaked up behind her and said boo.

Encourage each child to show how Carlos would feel if he were playing with a toy and April took it away.

Spinning Wheel

Help children make emotions wheels that are divided into sections for happy, sad, mad, scared and any other emotions they want. These are complex drawings, so you may want to have stickers for children to place on the wheels.

Each wheel should have the child's name on it. Wheels should be displayed where children can reach them and identify their own. Throughout the day, children can change the arrow as their feelings change. Encourage children to use words also to tell how they feel.

Brainstorming

Ask children to list ways people show they care about each other or about pets.

Show You Care

Have children choose a way to let someone at school know they care about him or her. At the end of the day, ask if children did something for this person. Let them tell what they did.

Allow time during the day for children to make something for someone they care about at home. Remind children to take their gifts home to show their special someone that they care.

Traditional Learning Centers
. . . .

Art

Add pictures of people looking happy, sad, angry, fearful and loving.

Housekeeping

Increase the number of mirrors.

Manipulative

Include games and puzzles relating to emotions.

Resources

* *

More information on these resources can be found starting on p. 261.

Books

Love and Happiness
Apple Pie and Onions
Ask Mr. Bear
The Giving Tree
Hold My Hand
A Little Book of Love
The Quarreling Book
Watch Out for the Chicken
   Feet in Your Soup
Will I Have a Friend?

Anger
Alexander and the Terrible,
   Horrible, No Good, Very
   Bad Day
I'm Mad at You
Let's Be Enemies

Sadness
Moving Day
William's Doll

Fear
Ira Sleeps Over
There's a Nightmare in My
   Closet
Where the Wild Things Are

Other Emotions
Grownups Cry Too
I Have Feelings

Songs

Love and Happiness
Baby Beluga
   All I Really Need
Circle Around
   Hug Bug
   Magic Penny
   Tickle Tune Typhoon Theme
Everything Grows
   Teddy Bear Hug
Hug the Earth
   Hug the Earth
Peace Is the World Smiling
   Peace Is the World Smiling

Fear
Circle Around
   Bear Hunt
   Sneakers
Free to Be ... a Family
   I'm Never Afraid
Sing Your Sillies Out
   The Wind

Anger
Free to Be ... a Family
   It's Not My Fault
   The Stupid Song

Here We Go...Watch Me Grow!

Sadness
And One and Two
  Good Day Everybody
Sing Your Sillies Out
  Blues Away

Other Emotions
All of Us Will Shine
  Let's Be Friends
  There Is a Fine Wind Blowing
Everything Grows
  Teddy Bear Hug
Free to Be...a Family
  Another Cinderella
Hug the Earth
  If You're Happy

Peace Is the World Smiling
  Find a Peaceful Thought
  Kid's Peace Song
  Make Peace
  Peace Dove
Sing Your Sillies Out
  Blues Away
  Funny Bone Rag
Teaching Peace
  I Think You're Wonderful
  Say Hi!
  Teaching Peace
Voyage for Dreamers
  Many the Flowers
  When Nighttime Sweeps the Land

Poems, Rhymes and Fingerplays

Love and Happiness
Where the Sidewalk Ends
  Hug O'War
  Love

Fear
Where the Sidewalk Ends
  Afraid of the Dark

Other
Finger Frolics
  When I Am ...

Free to Be ... a Family
  I'll Fix Anthony
  In My Room
  It's Not My Fault
  Some Things Don't Make Any Sense at All
Where the Sidewalk Ends
  Magical Eraser
  What a Day

Objective 4
What I Like About Myself

*Children will be able to identify characteristics
they like about themselves.*

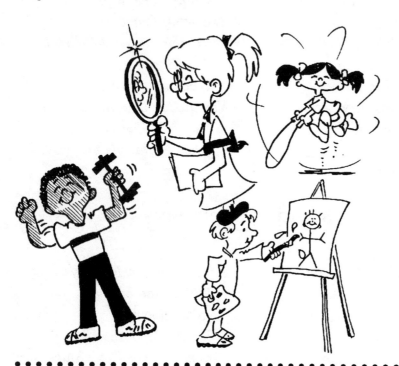

The purpose of this objective is to help children develop
self-confidence and high self-esteem. Children can recognize characteristics about themselves that they like or of
which they are proud.

Such characteristics may include physical characteristics—eye or hair color or height. They may also include
developmental skills—the ability to run fast, catch a ball,
jump rope or work puzzles; language/art skills—the ability
to read, draw, color or sing; and social/nurturing skills—the
ability to make friends, help at home or take care of pets.

62

Use these activities throughout the year to help children recognize and remember these characteristics.

Activities ....

Surveys

Survey children to find out what they like about themselves. Write down each child's name and response.

Circle Share

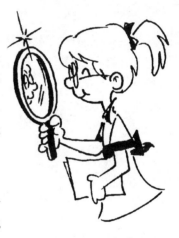

Encourage children to tell what they like about themselves. You should also tell something you like about yourself.

Tell all the children something you really like about each child (what makes each one special).

Language Experience Story

Encourage children to tell a story about something they're good at. Suggest that children begin by saying, "I am really good at...."

Movie Time

Make a videotape of all the children. Let each child select something to do or say in the movie. Play it back for all the children to see. Make an extra copy to loan to families with video viewing equipment.

Me

Encourage children to make books about themselves. Children can cut out pictures and dictate stories for you to write for them. Take a picture of each child to include in the book. Pictures can show activities children like to do and do well (such as running, singing, etc.).

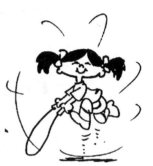

Make a Puzzle

Take a picture of each child. Help children cut the pictures into puzzle pieces. Children will be more successful in putting the puzzle together if you limit the number of pieces they cut. Store the puzzles in envelopes.

Proud Sticker

Discuss what being proud of yourself means. Give examples of things you are proud of. Print one of these things on a blank sticker. (A name badge or address label will work.) Ask children to tell you something they are proud of. Write what they tell you on a sticker for each child.

Tell Another

Have children choose partners. Partners tell each other something they like about the other. All children change partners and tell their new partners something they like about them. The game continues in this way.

Do not force children to say things they don't mean. Don't make children feel guilty if they don't like anything about another child. Let the other child tell what he or she likes about him- or herself, or you can tell what you like about the child. Demonstrate this game before the children play it by asking them to tell things they like about Kevin, April, Carlos and Mieko.

Notes from Home

Send home a form asking family members to write down what they like about their children. Read the comments to the children. If positive responses are not available for every child (for example, a parent forgot to complete the form), find another adult to complete a form for those children without one.

Traditional Learning Centers

Art

Provide a specific area and tape so children can hang their own work when they choose.

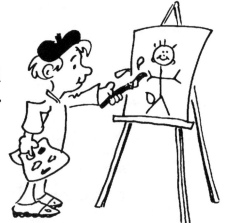

Blocks

Provide a camera so children can take pictures of their structures.

Housekeeping

Add more mirrors of all sizes and different shapes. Make the camera available to take pictures during house play.

Manipulative

Arrange a saving space for children to display creations made in the manipulative center.

Resources
· ·

More information on these resources can be found starting on p. 261.

Books

A Bird Can Fly

Cornelius

Crafty Chameleon

Green Eggs and Ham

I Know I'm Myself Because

Just Like Me

Swimmy

Yertle the Turtle and Other
  Stories

You Look Ridiculous

Songs

All of Us Will Shine
  East / West
    Everyone Is Differently Abled
    My Body Belongs to Me
Everything Grows
  Ha Ha Thisaway
  Little White Duck
Free to Be ... a Family
  Free to Be ... a Family
  Yourself Belongs to You

Hug the Earth
  Super Kids
Sing Your Sillies Out
  You Are a Star
Teaching Peace
  See Me Beautiful
When My Shoes Are Loose
  When My Shoes Are Loose

Poems, Rhymes and Fingerplays

Finger Frolics
  Me
  My Arms

Objective 5
Feeling Sad

Children will be able to explain that it is okay to feel sad when someone or something dies.

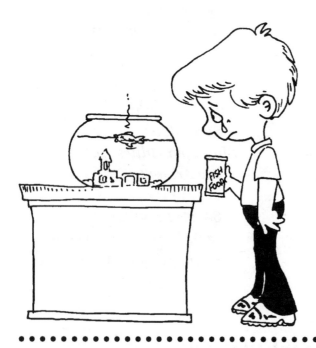

The purpose of this objective is to help children understand that death is a natural event and that sadness about death is normal. The timing of this objective is flexible. It may be used when and if a child in the class experiences the death of a family member, friend, classmate or pet. However, it may be easier to approach this concept when there has *not* been a recent death related to a class member.

The questions children ask will let you know how much you need to discuss about death. Remember that often you must talk with children individually about death.

Preschool age children do not view death as final, but believe there is a chance the person or pet will return. Help children view death as a normal occurrence rather than a frightening one. Discourage the use of phrases such as gone to sleep, gone away or gone on a trip.

Expose children to different beliefs about death. Be sensitive to the fact that families have different values related to death. Beliefs and values are often rooted in various cultural and religious backgrounds.

Your attitudes will be apparent to children, so evaluate your own feelings. Be sure you're able to deal with the topic yourself before trying to help children deal with it.

Activities •

Classroom Guests

Invite a guest to visit and talk to the children about why people have funerals. Look for people with various ideas about funerals, so children can hear how different people feel. Caution guests to talk at the level of preschoolers and to *comfort* the children and to take care not to scare them.

Brainstorming

Ask children to list ways people can help others feel better.

Field Trips

Take a field trip to a cemetery. Read the markers and tombstones. Make rubbings of the markers or tombstones by placing paper over the words and letting children rub the paper with a crayon. Look at different kinds of flowers. Take some flowers to leave either for someone the children knew or for a place without flowers.

Examination

Examine a dead (stuffed/preserved) animal. Allow children to look closely. If it is a stuffed animal, allow children to touch it. If a stuffed animal is not available, use a dead insect. For health reasons, it is not advisable for children to touch a dead insect. Children can tell about experiences seeing or touching a dead person or animal.

Sympathy Cards

Read a variety of sympathy cards to children. Discuss the meaning and purpose of the cards. Let children look at the pictures and words. As appropriate, encourage children to make sympathy cards.

Funerals

Tell children about funerals and the purpose of funerals. Explain that funerals help comfort the living people and show respect for the person who has died. Be sensitive to various cultural and religious beliefs.

Flower Arrangements

Let children arrange artificial flowers in different ways. Explain that when someone dies, people may send flowers to the family. Note that instead of flowers, some families ask that money be given to a charity or other organizations. This money might be used to help doctors learn more about diseases so others can live longer.

Vocabulary

Introduce and explain the words *dead* and *die*.

Why

Help children understand that death is natural and everyone dies sometime. Some people die because they are very old; some people are sick; or some may have been in accidents.

Breathe

Have all the children take deep breaths and use their hands to feel their stomachs push out as they breathe in. Have children breathe in and then blow air out their mouths. Explain that when someone dies, that person does not breathe anymore.

Obituaries

Read a few obituaries from a newspaper to children. Explain that these people have died. Explain words such as *survived by* or other words they may not understand.

Life Cycle

Show the children a seed, a healthy plant and a dead plant. Discuss the plant life cycle. Explain that people are born, they grow and they die.

Leaves

Bring in green leaves, some wilted leaves and some dry and brittle leaves. Encourage children to explore the likenesses and differences. Let children crumble the dead leaves. Explain that dead leaves become part of the earth.

Traditional Learning Centers

Housekeeping

Add artificial flowers for children to arrange and rear-range.

Science

Add nonpoisonous plants in various stages of life and death for children to examine and care for.

Resources

More information on these resources can be found starting on p. 261.

Books

*About Dying: An Open Family
    Book for Parents and
    Children Together*
The Dead Bird
Everett Anderson's Goodbye
My Grandpa Died Today

My Grandson Lew
*The Tenth Good Thing About
    Barney*
The Velveteen Rabbit
Will It Be Okay?

Songs

Singable Songs
    Five Little Frogs
Sing Your Sillies Out
    The Watermelon Song

When My Shoes Are Loose
    I'm Just Hungry
    Worms

Poems, Rhymes and Fingerplays

Finger Frolics
  The Falling Star

Objective 6
Social Behavior

Children will be able to identify appropriate and inappropriate social behavior.

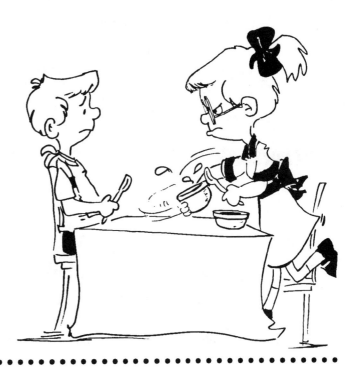

The purpose of this objective is to help children learn appropriate and inappropriate behavior for a variety of social situations. Provide activities to help children learn basic social skills. General classroom management and school rules also help teach appropriate social behavior.

Encourage children to use the words *please, thank you* and *excuse me*. Social manners to teach include appropriate table manners, not interrupting when someone else is talking and sharing with others.

When teaching children to share, encourage children to take turns and share toys, but do not always expect young children to give up favored items. Be sure you have realistic expectations for children regarding other behaviors, such as following rules.

Practice activities that encourage appropriate social behavior throughout the year. Appropriate behavior is also taught by modeling for children. Everything you do and say sends a message to children.

Activities . . . .

Roleplay

Give each child a turn to show what Carlos would do if he were playing with a toy and Mieko took it away.

Encourage each child to show what Kevin would do if he wanted a toy April was playing with.

Circle Share

Ask each child, "How do you feel when someone says *please* to you?"

Problem Solving

Describe a situation and ask children what they think they could do in that situation. Encourage several answers, and help children see that there is usually more than one right way. Examples: What could you do if...?

- Your mother says you can't have any cookies, but you want some.

- Your mother says you can't have any cookies, but you sneak and get some anyway and the jar breaks.

- Your grandmother has gone outside in the garden and told you not to answer the telephone. It rings and rings.

- Your daddy told you to stay in the house and that he would be right back. He is next door, and a fire starts in your house.

- You want to play with a toy someone else is playing with.

- Someone is standing in your way on the sidewalk.

- A friend says something to you, and you can't hear everything he or she said.

- You bump into someone, but it is an accident.

- Your sister gives you a toy.

- The food you want is on the other side of the table, and you can't reach it.

- Someone knocks down the blocks you were building with.

Brainstorming

Ask children why Carlos, Kevin, April and Mieko need *rules* at school.

Ask children when Kevin should say *please*. Examples: if he wants April to listen to him, if he wants a toy Carlos is playing with, etc.

Ask children when April should say *thank you*. Examples: if Mieko lets April play with her toy, if a relative gives her a present, if a teacher tells her he or she likes her shoes, etc.

Brainstorm polite words such as *please, thank you, you're welcome.*

Rules

Make up a few class rules. Older preschool children can help make rules. Write, illustrate and display these rules. Use positive language (walk down the hall) instead of negative (do not run in the hall).

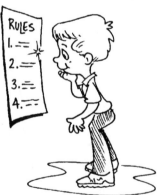

Demonstrate how to follow the rules. Gently remind children as needed. Young children forget and may have difficulty understanding rules. Model the rules by your own actions.

Traditional Learning Centers ....

Art

Draw step-by-step directions for painting or any other messy activity. Explain the directions to the children, and display the directions for ongoing use.

Blocks

Label the block shelf with outlines of each type of unit block to show where blocks should be returned after use. Paper or felt can be used for the outlines.

Housekeeping

Place the pots, pans and dishes on contact paper. Trace around them and cut the contact paper on the lines. Apply the contact paper to the shelves or walls where the containers should be returned after use.

Manipulative

Add trays or place mats for children to use when working a puzzle or playing with another manipulative item. When children confine their space to a visible area like a place mat, they learn to respect each other's space and projects.

Resources ●

More information on these resources can be found starting on p. 261.

Books

Everybody Takes Turns

I Can't Wait

I Want It

Little Witch's Big Night

May I?

My Name Is Not Dummy

Songs

And One and Two
  Good Day Everybody
  Sharing
Baby Beluga
  Thanks a Lot
  To Everyone in All the World
Everything Grows
  Little White Duck
Free to Be ... a Family
  The Stupid Song
  Thank Someone
Learning Basic Skills
  Cover Your Mouth
  Keep the Germs Away
  Take a Bath
Peace Is the World Smiling
  Make Peace
Singable Songs
  Five Little Frogs
  Robin in the Rain
  The Sharing Song

Sing Your Sillies Out
  Cooperate
  Funny Bone Rag
Teaching Peace
  Say Hi!
  Shake Your Brains
  Teaching Peace
  Use a Word
  With Two Wings
Travellin' with Ella Jenkins
  Greetings in Many Languages
  Thank You in Several
    Languages
When My Shoes Are Loose
  I'm Just Hungry
  Legs, Slow Down
  When My Shoes Are Loose
  Would You Please

Poems, Rhymes and Fingerplays

Finger Frolics
  Being Kind
  Manners
  Please and Thank You
  Table Manners
  Thumbkin
Free to Be ... a Family
  Thank Someone

Where the Sidewalk Ends
  I'm Making a List
  Pancake?
  Ridiculous Rose
  Tight Hat

3.

Personal Health

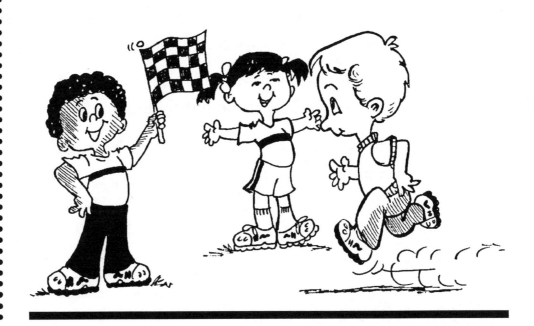

Personal Health

During the preschool years, children develop health habits, both healthful and harmful. This unit promotes development of *healthy* (positive) habits in the areas of grooming, exercise and other personal health practices. Such healthy behavior will help maintain the body and promote overall wellness (feeling good).

Lifestyle Goals

Successful completion of this curriculum will put children on the road to achieving lifelong goals of:

- developing and adhering to a lifestyle that promotes personal well-being;

- pursuing leisure-time activities that promote physical fitness and relieve mental and emotional tension;

- following health-care practices that prevent illness and maintain health.

Objective 7
When You're Hurt

Children will be able to name an appropriate person to tell if they hurt physically or emotionally.

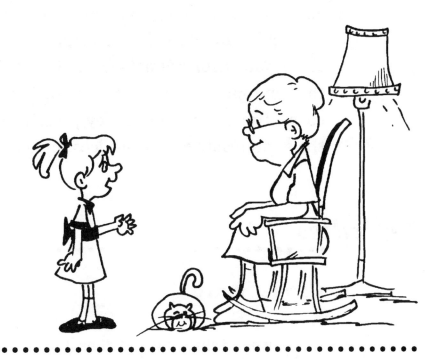

The purpose of this objective is to teach children to contact a responsible adult, rather than telling a friend their age or keeping a secret, if they are either physically or emotionally hurt.

Discuss what it feels like to be physically hurt. Explain the importance of doing what is needed to get well. Stress the importance of being honest and not playing sick or hurt to stay home or get your way.

Discuss what it feels like to have your feelings hurt. Explain the importance of doing what is needed, such as talking to someone, to feel better. Stress the importance of being honest about your feelings and not playing hurt to get your way.

The child's hurt may involve such situations as falling down, being called names by other children, or abuse or neglect by an adult. If you suspect child abuse or neglect, check your agency's policies and procedures to determine the appropriate course of action. If such policies do not currently exist in your agency, preschool or daycare, contact the appropriate social services in your area for advice.

Activities

Circle Share

Ask each child, "What does it mean to have your feelings hurt?" Ask children who they should tell if their feelings are hurt.

Roleplay

Encourage each child to act like a part of his or her body is hurting.

Brainstorming

Encourage children to name grown-ups they could tell if they were hurt.

Brainstorm characters in television shows or movies who have been hurt (such as a cartoon character, someone who is hurt in an accident, etc.). Discuss how they were helped or how they could (or should) ask for help.

Collages

Let children make a group collage of pictures of people who are hurt, such as a person using crutches or with a bandage. Be careful that the pictures do not depict violent situations that may upset the children.

Language Experience Story

Encourage each child to tell an experience story about being hurt. Help children begin by saying, "Once when I was hurt...," and let them finish the sentence.

Classroom Guests

Invite a mental health professional to visit the classroom and tell the children about his or her job. Explain to children that some people tell the counselor when their feelings are hurt.

Problem Solving

Describe the following situations and ask the children what Mieko should do. Ask children if there are other things Mieko could do. What could Mieko do if...?

- She fell off the swing and hurt her leg. Her leg hurts when she tries to walk.

- She sees April fall off the slide.

- Her stomach hurts and she feels like crying.

- Someone keeps hugging her and won't let go. She doesn't want the person to hug her.

- Someone she really loves hits her and hurts her.

Ask children to describe what they think will happen when they tell a grown-up that they hurt. Help children see that different grown-ups may respond in different ways. Some grown-ups may not listen, and others may pay close attention. Some grown-ups may get help from a doctor or counselor.

Breathing

Encourage children to practice deep breathing. Tell them to take a breath and push their stomachs out. Then show children how to blow air out and make their stomachs get smaller. Explain that slow, deep breathing helps people when they hurt.

Traditional Learning Centers

Housekeeping

Add first-aid supplies such as bandages, Band-Aids, body lotion, etc., to play with.

Manipulative

Include puzzles of hospitals and families.

Resources

More information on these resources can be found starting on p. 261.

Books

The Boy Who Cried Wolf
Chicken Little
Chilly Stomach
Samit and the Dragon

Sheila Rae, the Brave
The Surprise Party
Talking Without Words
Wellin Magic

Songs

Free to Be ... a Family
  I'm Never Afraid
  Yourself Belongs to You

Singable Songs
  Spider on the Floor

Sing Your Sillies Out
Blues Away
Voyage for Dreamers
After the Rain Falls

When My Shoes Are Loose
Telephone
Would You Please

Poems, Rhymes and Fingerplays

Finger Frolics
Caring for an Abrasion
Free to Be ... a Family
I'm Never Afraid (to Say
What's on My Mind)

Where the Sidewalk Ends
Sick

Objective 8
Brush Your Teeth

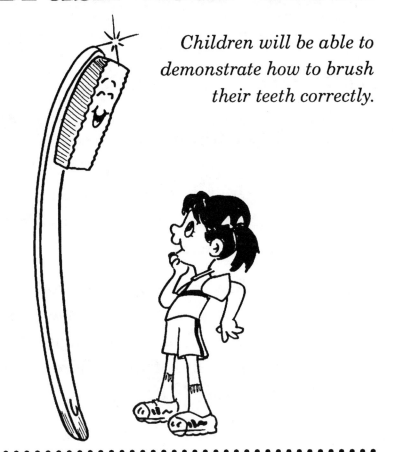

Children will be able to demonstrate how to brush their teeth correctly.

The purpose of this objective is to help children recognize the importance of brushing teeth and practice correct techniques for brushing.

Stress the importance of brushing *correctly,* because many children may not yet have the ability to brush their teeth on all surfaces. If they learn the correct technique and the importance of it, they are more likely to brush properly when their motor coordination becomes sufficiently developed.

Some children may not have toothbrushes and toothpaste at home. Local dental offices or stores may be willing to donate these supplies.

Activities

Big Choppers

Use a large model of teeth and gums to demonstrate correct brushing techniques. You may want to show only one step each day.

Show and emphasize that children should wiggle the toothbrush. Have children wiggle all over. Show them how to hold the brush at an angle against the base of the tooth and gum line. Have children imagine they are holding a toothbrush at an angle.

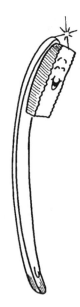

Show children how they should wiggle in a circular motion and sweep to the end of the tooth. Ask children to imagine and try wiggling and sweeping their brush. This applies to both outer and inner surfaces.

Show children how to scrub against biting surfaces of chewing teeth. Ask children to imagine and try. Let different children demonstrate with the big teeth. The model may also be left out during learning center time for all children to practice with.

Tablets

Obtain disclosing tablets from a dentist or drugstore, and read the directions. Explain to children that the tablets will leave red spots on their teeth. The spots indicate areas of plaque that need to be brushed a lot.

Let children chew the tablets and examine their teeth with mirrors. Encourage children to brush until all the red spots are gone. Send a note home to inform parents or other adults about the activity.

Mouthwash

Show children several different mouthwashes. Read a little of each bottle's label to the children. Demonstrate how to swish mouthwash without swallowing it. Let each child try the mouthwash. Select a mouthwash that does not contain alcohol. You may want to choose one with fluoride.

Floss

Demonstrate how to use dental floss. Explain that people use floss, in addition to brushing, to keep the spaces between teeth clean.

Water Spray

Show children dental water-spray devices and explain that these devices help clean between teeth. Let each child spray water into the sink or another container.

Explain that children cannot take turns spraying in their mouths for two reasons. One is that the dentist didn't recommend they use a water spray. The other is that there are not separate sprayers for each child, and it is unhealthy to put something in your mouth that has been in someone else's mouth.

Swish

Explain that when you can't brush, you should at least put water in your mouth, swish it and swallow it. Let the children try this.

Decay Experiment

Get two apples with no bad spots or bruises. Make a hole in the skin on one apple—use a pencil or other sharp object. Tell children what you are going to do and ask them what they think will happen. Then let them help. Observe the apples daily to see what happens. (The one with the hole will rot faster, and the hole will get bigger.)

Classroom Guests

Invite a dentist or dental assistant to visit the class and teach about tooth care.

Fluoride Experiment

In a small group, explain that you are going to conduct an experiment. Show children the word *fluoride*. Let them find the word on various toothpaste containers. Explain that fluoride is a mineral that helps teeth to be strong. It also helps protect our teeth against cavities (holes).

Fluoride is usually in the drinking water and in most toothpastes. Explain that dentists can put extra fluoride on teeth if they think you need more.

Hold up two boiled eggs, and tell the children you are going to conduct an experiment using the eggs. Let the children watch you paint one egg with fluoride but not the other egg. Ask which egg they think will be stronger. Remind them about using fluoride on their teeth.

Have two containers and label one of them *fluoride*. Let children pour vinegar into each container. Place the egg that was painted into the container with the fluoride label and the other egg into the other container.

Ask children what they think will happen. Watch what happens. Leave the containers out and check them throughout the day. Explain to children that their teeth are like the eggs. Their teeth will stay strong if they take care of them.

Check It

Create a chart with the children's names on it. Let children place a check by their name when they brush their teeth.

Cut It

Give each child a plastic knife. Provide a variety of foods for the children to cut. After cutting the food, examine the knife to see if there are any remains of food on it or if it appears to be clean. Explain that foods that stick to the knife also stick to teeth. Some foods to test are marshmallows, honey, cake and fruits.

Check the Teeth

Using either a comb for each child or the large teeth model, have children stick the teeth of the comb or the model into various substances. Then brush the teeth to see which foods are easy to remove and which ones are difficult. Try using syrup, honey and marshmallows for the sticky substances and mashed potatoes and milk for nonsticky ones.

Practice

Arrange the daily schedule to include a time for children to brush their teeth. Use the big teeth model to reinforce the way children should brush. Also arrange time for the older children to use dental floss. Remember, children learn through modeling, so brush and floss your teeth, too.

Special Learning Centers

Dentist's Office

Set up a special area for the dentist to examine patients. Include a flashlight, mirror and dentist's coat. Place pictures of teeth around the office.

Traditional Learning Centers

Art

Add brushes of various sizes and shapes.

Housekeeping

Add empty containers for toothpaste, mouthwash and dental floss.

Science

Add several kinds of toothbrushes for children to examine. Remind children to look at the brushes, but *not* to put the brushes in their mouths.

Resources •

More information on these resources can be found starting on p. 261.

Books

Albert's Toothache
The Alligator's Toothache
How Many Teeth?
Little Rabbit's Loose Tooth

My Dentist
Our Tooth Story: A Tale of
   Twenty-two Teeth
Teeth

Songs

All of Us Will Shine
   Pearly White Waltz
Learning Basic Skills
   Brush Away
   Keep the Germs Away

Singable Songs
   Brush Your Teeth

Poems, Rhymes and Fingerplays

Finger Frolics
   Brushing Teeth
   Getting Dressed
   This Is the Way We...

Where the Sidewalk Ends
   Wild Boar

Objective 9
What to Wear

Children will be able to identify appropriate clothing for different weather conditions.

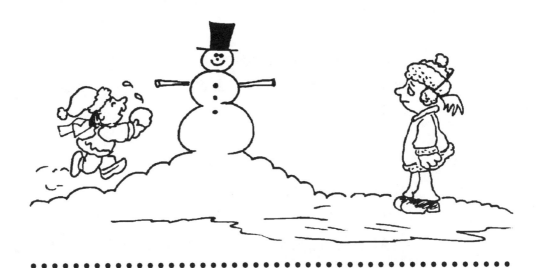

The purpose of this objective is to help children select clothing appropriate for different weather conditions. It also helps children see the importance of clothing for health and safety.

Appropriate clothing should be selected for weather or other environmental conditions. Heavy clothes in the winter help keep us warm and may help prevent illness.

These concepts can be introduced and taught during one unit. However, they should be emphasized at the beginning of each season and other appropriate times.

Activities ••

Discovery Box

Place various 11-inch fashion doll clothes in the box. Let children pull out one outfit at a time and tell if the clothes should be worn when it is hot, cold, raining, snowing, etc.

Roleplay

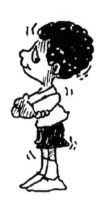

Suggest that children act like it is raining (or snowing, hot, cold, etc.) and they are outside.

Paper People

At the beginning of each season, draw the outline of each child again. Let children paint or color clothes appropriate for that season on their paper people.

Collages

Let children make a group collage of winter clothes on one half of the page and summer clothes on the other half.

Mobiles

Encourage children to make mobiles of things relating to a season of the year.

Dressed for Nighttime

Turn the lights off, and use a flashlight to see who is most safely dressed for nighttime walking. Point out that wearing lightly colored clothes makes it easier for others to see us at night.

One Season

Obtain pictures of places where the temperature is fairly constant, for example, Hawaii or Florida. Show children the pictures and tell them about the weather there.

Lotto

Make a lotto game with pictures of hats, and encourage children to play it. Tell children that covering their heads when it is cold is very important, because it helps keep the rest of the body warm.

Walks

Take a walk and look for things unique to the season. In the spring you may find flower or tree-leaf buds. Colorful fallen leaves may be examined in autumn.

Where Does It Go?

Have clothes from all seasons. Encourage children to place the clothes in a box with a sun on it or a box with snow or rain, depending on when the clothes should be worn.

Traditional Learning Centers

Art

Add pictures representing different seasons.

Blocks

Add cotton to be used for snow and small flower and tree accessories. Post pictures of structures during different seasons.

Housekeeping

Add dress-up clothes of different seasons. Include many textures. (We do not recommend hats because they can spread head lice.) Put place mats that represent different seasons on the table. Add doll clothes to represent different seasons.

Manipulative

Include puzzles showing different seasons. Add a doll house and dolls with clothes for different seasons.

Science

Add ice for children to handle and observe.

Resources

···

More information on these resources can be found starting on p. 261.

Books

Gilberto and the Wind
Growing Story
The Snowman
The Snowy Day

Spring Is Here
Stopping by Woods on a
  Snowy Evening
A Tree Is Nice

Songs

Everything Grows
  Just Like the Sun
  Mary Wore Her Red Dress
One Light, One Sun
  Mr. Sun

Singable Songs
  Robin in the Rain
When My Shoes Are Loose
  Every Year I Have a Birthday
  When My Shoes Are Loose

Poems, Rhymes and Fingerplays

Finger Frolics
  Blowing Bubbles
  Burr-rr-rr
  Climatology
  Dress for the Weather
  Eensy Weensy Spider
  Getting Dressed
  I Godda Code
  My Zipper Suit

The Rainbow
Signs of Autumn
Warm Hands
Weather
The Wind
Where the Sidewalk Ends
  Rain
  Snowman

104

Objective 10
Exercise Helps Us Grow

Children will be able to list ways that exercise helps our bodies grow and develop properly.

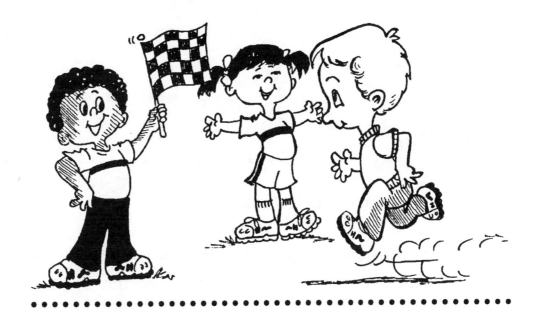

The purpose of this objective is to make children aware of the benefits of regular exercise. Most young children enjoy running, jumping and other forms of exercise. Therefore, this is an appropriate time to develop healthy exercise habits.

Exercise is helpful in many ways. We can see some of the ways it helps, such as developing strong arms and legs, or being able to run a long distance without getting tired. Exercise also helps inside our bodies by making our bones, muscles and heart strong.

Encourage children to exercise regularly. Any kind of exercise is good, but exercise is most helpful if it is continuous exercise. For example, running, jumping rope or riding tricycles involves *continuous* movement.

Activities such as playing T-ball aren't as beneficial, because children hit the ball and run, but then stop running until it is their turn again. Such start/stop activities are not as helpful in building strong hearts.

Emphasize that exercise can be fun if we do things we enjoy.

Activities

Classroom Guests

Invite a guest who exercises regularly. Tell children that everyone needs to take care of him- or herself. Ask the guest to lead the children in some warm-up exercises, if appropriate.

Invite an aerobics teacher to come and demonstrate aerobic exercise or dance. Ask him or her to teach the children a few simple activities.

Invite a bicyclist, runner, swimmer or other athlete to talk to the children about his or her sport.

Field Trips

Take a field trip to a health club or fitness center. Look at the exercise equipment and weights. Ask for demonstrations of the equipment. If appropriate, let the children try out the equipment. Tour the center to see if there are other health facilities such as a sauna, whirlpool, racquetball courts, etc.

Daily Schedule

Arrange the daily schedule to include an exercise time. Exercise with the children to model positive health habits.

Walks

Take the class for a walk for the health of it. Walk briskly and record how far and how long you walk. Explain that some people walk for exercise.

Surveys

Have children survey people in your building to see if they exercise regularly (three times a week or more). Ask those who do exercise what type of exercise they do and why they exercise. Also survey family members to see if they exercise regularly. Ask if

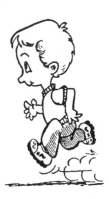

they exercise at work, as recreation (such as sports or hiking) or in an exercise program.

Brainstorming

Brainstorm the different ways people exercise.

Yoga

Introduce the children to yoga to show ways to exercise and increase flexibility through proper stretching exercises.

Special Learning Centers

Bodybuilding

Set up an exercise center where children can strengthen their bodies through exercise. Add a mat to an area away from traffic. Display pictures of people exercising. Add exercise records and/or videotapes if appropriate.

Traditional Learning Centers

Art

Place large strips of paper (newsprint or butcher paper) on the wall from the floor to above the children's heads. Provide paint. Children will need to stretch and bend to paint the paper. Tape paper under the tables for children to color on. They will need to lie on their backs and reach up.

Housekeeping

Add exercise clothing and accessories.

Science

Add wrist weights and small hand weights to weigh in balance scales.

Resources

More information on these resources can be found starting on p. 261.

Books

Be a Frog, a Bird or a Tree:
   Carr's Creative Yoga
   Exercises for Children
Bill and Pete
Bunnies and Their Sports

Calico Cat's Exercise Book
Happy, Healthy Pooh Book
Human Body Book
The Longest Journey in the
   World

Loudmouth George and the
  Big Race
See What I Can Do: A Book of
  Creative Movement

Yoga for Children

Songs

All of Us Will Shine
  East / West
  Hokey Pokey
And One and Two
  And One and Two
  Jumping with Variations
  Marching to Harmonica
    Melody
  Rhythms Round the Chair
Baby Beluga
  Baby Beluga
  Joshua Giraffe
Circle Around
  Clap Your Hands
  Muscle Music
  Sneakers
  Tree Dancin'
  Vega Boogie

Everything Grows
  Brown Girl in the Ring
Hug the Earth
  Doin' the Robot
  Knickerbocker
  Kye Kye Kule
Learning Basic Skills
  Exercise Every Day
  Posture Exercises
One Light, One Sun
  The Bowling Song
  Tingalayo
Sing Your Sillies Out
  Shake Your Sillies Out
  Someone's in the Middle
  Use Your Own Two Feet
When My Shoes Are Loose
  How the Animals Go

Poems, Rhymes and Fingerplays

Finger Frolics
  Getting Dressed
  If I Were a Horse
  Little Huey Dragon
  My Little Tricycle

  Not Say a Single Word
  Stretch up High
Where the Sidewalk Ends
  Dancing Pants
  Lazy Jane

4.

Family Life and Health

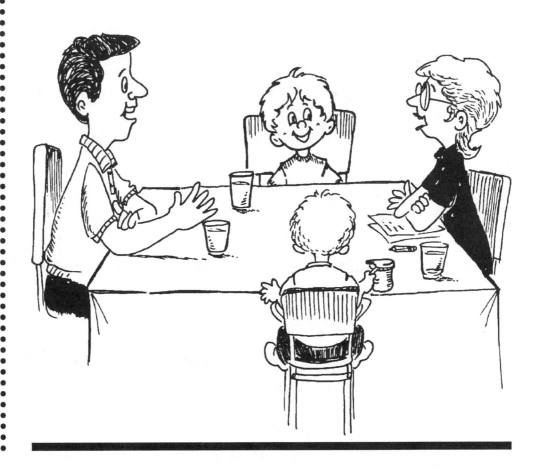

Family Life and Health

This unit explores the roles and interactions of individuals within the family life cycle. Each family member has certain responsibilities. Family members may also have different privileges based on age or maturity. Each person experiences physical, mental and social changes. The family unit (mother, father, stepparent, aunt or uncle, etc.) is responsible for helping children mature both physically and socially.

Lifestyle Goals

Successful completion of this curriculum will put children on the road to achieving lifelong goals of:

- identifying and respecting the rights and privileges of every family member;

- adjusting appropriately to changing physical, mental and social roles, responsibilities and privileges as they occur throughout the life cycle;

- dealing comfortably and appropriately with the demands of their genders;

- supporting the belief that the health of all children is an individual, family and community responsibility.

Objective 11
Helping at Home

*Children will be able to identify
ways to help at home.*

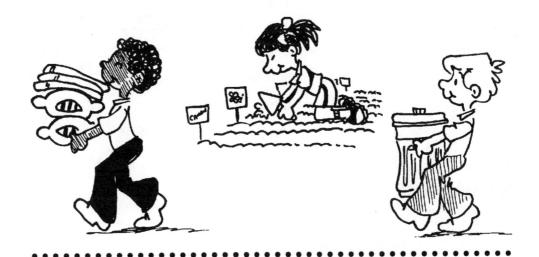

. . . .

The purpose of this objective is to emphasize individual responsibility within the family. There are two ideas which should be emphasized. First, children can identify what needs to be done at home. Second, children can identify what they can do to help.

For example: If dishes need to be washed, children may be able to help by drying the forks and spoons and putting them away. Children may be too young to wash breakable plates and drinking glasses, but they might wash plastic dishes and cups.

Activities may be done inside or outside the house. Outside tasks can include sweeping walkways, planting flowers, filling bird feeders or watering the garden. Inside tasks may include dusting, folding clothes, making the bed, and cleaning or setting the table. Allow children to do some of these activities in the classroom, such as cleaning the table, and encourage them to do so at home.

Encourage children to think about other ways they can help at home. For example: A child could help with younger children and new babies. The responsibility of caring for younger children may help develop some positive sibling bonding.

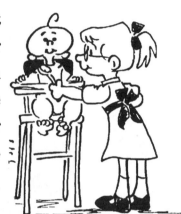

Activities

Brainstorming

Ask children to list ways people can help others. You may need to give children some classroom and home examples.

Where Does It Go?

Have pictures of people helping and pictures of other situations where people are not helping someone. Ask children to sort the pictures into a helping box with a smile on it or a box with the word *no* on it for the others.

Do You or Don't You?

Have children sit in a circle. Explain that each family is different. What children do to help in each family may be different. Tell children you are going to ask some questions and if the answer is yes, they should stand up. Then ask the following questions:

Do you help take care of a pet?

Do you help by dressing yourself?

Do you help by setting the table?

Do others help you?

Do you wash clothes?

Do you put away your toys?

Do you put clothes away?

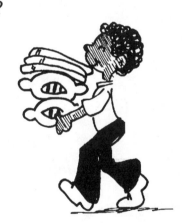

Helping Hands Tree

Make a "helping hands" tree. The tree can be a branch placed in a coffee can filled with rocks, a picture of a tree or any other representation of a tree. Children can help prepare the tree. When the tree is ready, follow this procedure:

Children choose something they can do at home to help a family member. To be sure the choice is acceptable at home, you may want to get several suggestions from the family of each child. Children then trace around one of their hands and cut out the tracing. (Children can cut out a circle or square around the handprint.)

Children tell you what they can do to help at home. Print whatever children say on their hands and read it to them. Children then attach their hands to the tree.

Children should share their experiences on the helping at home project from time to time. Send a note home explaining what the child is learning at school and the child's "helping hand" tracing.

Collages

Let children make a collage of magazine pictures of people helping other people.

Surveys

Have children ask people in the building what help is needed that children can provide. For example: Children may be able to help wipe the tables after lunch or pick up paper in the hallway and put it in the trash can.

Make appointments with individuals for children to ask what help is needed. Ask adults to tell the children and print it for the children. As a group, discuss the needs. Make plans to follow through on a few projects to be helpful.

Language Experience Story

Let each child tell an experience story about helping. Suggest stories about how it feels to help, how they help others or how others help them.

Traditional Learning Centers

Housekeeping

Help children make a chart to place on the refrigerator. List jobs that need to be done in the housekeeping center. Use pictures beside each word. The chart can have a place for children to write their names in when they volunteer. Be creative and make a different kind of chart each day.

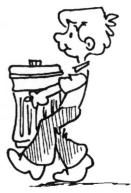

Science

Add a pet to the science center, and teach children how to care for it. Be sure to take the pet to a veterinarian before placing it in the classroom. Classroom pets can include fish, hamsters, guinea pigs, gerbils, frogs and ants.

Resources •••••••••••••••••••••••••••••••••

More information on these resources can be found starting on p. 261.

Books

Clifford's Good Deeds
Do You Know What I'll Do?
Howie Helps Himself
The Little Red Hen

May I Visit?
Messy Bessey's Closet
Mr. Grumpy's Motor Car

Songs

Everything Grows
   Bathtime
Hug the Earth
   Garbage Blues

Sing Your Sillies Out
   I Had a Rooster
   Pig in a Pen
When My Shoes Are Loose
   Pick It Up

Poems, Rhymes and Fingerplays

Finger Frolics
   Getting Dressed
   Hammer, Hammer, Hammer

Helping Dad
Polishing My Shoes
Where the Sidewalk Ends
   Helping

Objective 12
Family Members

Children will be able to describe different types of family structures.

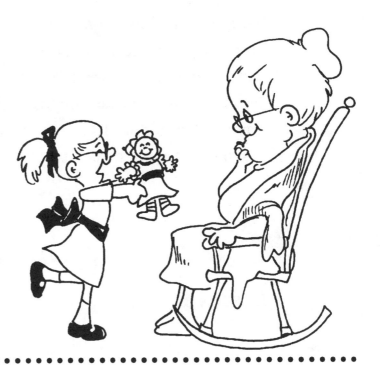

The purpose of this objective is to help children identify their own family members and roles and to recognize that there are different kinds of families. This objective should take several lessons.

Emphasize that no one family is just like another family. Include topics such as adoption, foster families, divorce, step-families and single-parent families in these discussions.

One of the best ways to teach that there are different kinds of families is not to assume that families are traditional. Take care not to say you are sending notes home to mothers. What about fathers, guardians, aunts, etc.? You could say instead that you are sending notes to the children's grown-ups or families. Display pictures of nontraditional families.

Aging may be discussed in this unit. Some children may have elderly relatives living with them, while other children may have limited exposure to older people. Children can realize that older people may have different ideas than the children are accustomed to. Also, some older people may have difficulty with vision or hearing. Children should learn how to interact with older people.

Activities

Discovery Box

Place pictures of individual people (may be magazine pictures) or small dolls in the Discovery Box. Let each child remove one and tell what family member it might be. On your turn (as teacher participant), suggest aunts, uncles, grandparents, cousins, stepparents, foster parents or other extended family members, so children will recognize various family structures.

Family Photo

Display photos of the children's families in the classroom. Encourage discussion.

Brainstorming

List television shows that have families on them. Discuss different kinds of families.

Classroom Guests

Invite an adoptive parent to share with the children about how he or she wanted to adopt a child. Invite an adult who was adopted and let him or her share that adoptive parents are a real family, too.

Invite a foster parent or social worker to explain what foster homes are and why they are important.

Invite a foster grandparent or other senior citizen to visit the classroom and tell about his or her family.

Circle Share

Ask children to share about their families. Help children by suggesting that they tell who is in their family.

Family Event

Plan a class-sponsored family event with the children. Let the children help decide if it will be a picnic, an open house or some other activity. Let children make the invitations and decorations. Prepare some of the food at school. Encourage every child to welcome every family.

House Building

In small groups, ask children to use blocks to build homes for families. Use 11-inch fashion dolls to show children the family they should build a house for. Suggest families with single parents, families that are ethnically mixed, large, divorced, extended, etc.

Explain that sometimes families don't all live together in the same house. Be prepared for children to ask why. Explain about foster families, blended families, divorced families and extended families.

Traditional Learning Centers

Art

Add different kinds of paper such as construction, typing and tissue paper. Help children understand these are all paper, even though they are different. Many kinds of paint, clay, crayons or markers can be added instead of paper.

Blocks

Add block accessory people representing different ages and ethnic groups.

Housekeeping

Add framed photographs of different families. Hang some on the wall and place others on tables or shelves. Find as many different kinds of families as possible. Be careful to use plastic rather than glass in the frames.

Manipulative

Add puppets representing different types of families. Add puzzles that represent different types of families.

Resources ••

More information on these resources can be found starting on p. 261.

Books

Abby
All Alone with Daddy
All Kinds of Families
Are You My Mother?
Big Sister and Little Sister
Black Is Brown Is Tan
Everett Anderson's Friend
A Father Like That
Free to Be ... a Family
Grandpa
Is That Your Sister?
Jenny Lives with Eric and Martin
Just Us Women
Kevin's Grandma
Make Way for Ducklings

Mom and Dad Don't Live Together Anymore
Mom Is Single
My Mom Travels a Lot
My Mother and I Are Growing Strong
New Life: New Room
On Mother's Lap
Peter's Chair
Rosie and Roo
She's Not My Real Mother
That New Baby
The Train
Where Is Daddy?
Your Family, My Family

Songs

Baby Beluga
  All I Really Need
  Over in the Meadow
Everything Grows
  Everything Grows
Free to Be ... a Family
  And Superboy Makes Three
  Another Cinderella
  Boy Meets Girl ... Again
  Free to Be ... a Family

Friendly Neighborhood
Something for Everyone
Some Things Don't Make Any Sense at All
Hug the Earth
  The Family Song
One Light, One Sun
  Down on Grandpa's Farm
Peace Is the World Smiling
  Make Peace

Here We Go...Watch Me Grow!

Poems, Rhymes and Fingerplays

Finger Frolics
  How Many...
Free to Be ... a Family
  Free to Be ... a Family
  Friendly Neighborhood
  Some Things Don't Make Any
    Sense at All

Where the Sidewalk Ends
  For Sale
  Two Boxes
  Upstairs

Objective 13
Family Jobs

Children will be able to list jobs of different family members.

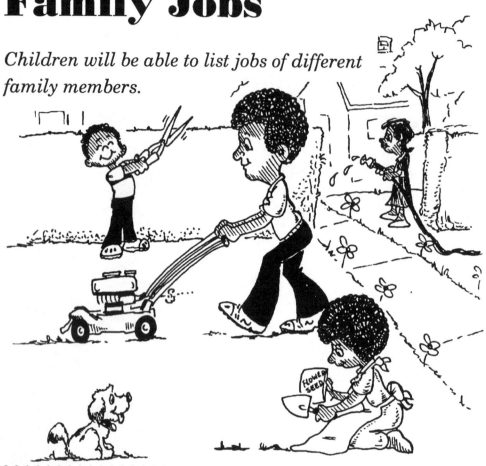

The purpose of this objective is to create awareness that family members have many different roles and responsibilities. Today's society requires different responsibilities of each member. Families must work together in whatever way is needed to maintain the family unit and to accomplish what needs to be done, regardless of gender.

In today's society, both men and women may be found taking responsibility for child care. Either or both parents may work outside the home to provide for the family. Household jobs such as washing dishes or laundry or taking

Here We Go...Watch Me Grow!

out the garbage are handled by either men or women, as is outside work, such as mowing the grass or building a porch.

Activities ··

Discovery Box

Place pictures of household jobs such as washing dishes, taking out the garbage, mowing the grass, planting flowers, etc., in the Discovery Box. As each child pulls out a picture, ask him or her to tell what the job is and who does it in his or her family.

Classroom Guests

Invite guests to tell the children what household jobs they do at home. Look for nontraditional families. Include single parents likely to be responsible for all household jobs.

Lotto

Make a household jobs lotto game to play with children. Include jobs inside the house and outside the house. Include jobs traditionally performed by males as well as those performed by females. Look for or make nontraditional pictures (such as a woman mowing the grass or a man washing dishes).

Spinning Wheel

Make a spinning wheel with pictures of household jobs that need to be done in the classroom. Washing the play dishes, taking out the trash, dusting, watering plants and other duties can be included. Let children spin and find out what their jobs will be in the classroom. If the arrow points to the same job twice, solve it in one of these ways:

- keep a chart for days to come;

- disregard the spin; or

- let children work together on the project.

Problem Solving

Ask children what would happen if each of the following occurred. Keep asking questions to help children identify the problems instead of just the logical answer.

- If no one washed the dishes, what would happen? (They would all be dirty.)

  Then what would happen? (The house might smell.)

  What else? (Bugs might come.)

  What else? (We wouldn't have dishes to eat on.)

- Other examples: What would happen if no one mowed the grass?

  What would happen if no one watered the plants?

What would happen if no one fixed the car when it was broken?

What would happen if no one washed clothes?

What would happen if no one bought food?

Roleplay

Ask all children (as a group) to act like they are taking out the trash, washing dishes, washing clothes, building a porch, grocery shopping, washing the floor, planting flowers, mowing the grass or other activities.

The Family Story

Introduce a nontraditional family of 11-inch fashion dolls to the children. Tell a story about the family. Give the dolls names and tell what household jobs they each have. Let children make up a family and story after you have finished.

Traditional Learning Centers ....

Art

Make a list of art jobs and assignments. Rotate assignments so that every child gets to do all the jobs. Sample jobs are wash brushes, wash table and check containers to be sure lids are on tight.

Housekeeping

Help children make a chart to place on the refrigerator. List jobs that need to be done in the housekeeping center. Use pictures beside each word. The chart can have a place for children to write their names in when they volunteer. Be creative and make a different kind of chart each day.

Manipulative

Add a doll house and dolls that can represent different family members.

Science

Add activities for identifying likenesses and differences. For example, add marbles for sorting by color and buttons to sort by color, size, shape and number of holes.

Resources ●

More information on these resources can be found starting on p. 261.

Books

Joshua's Day

Lots of Mommies

Love You Forever

Martin's Father

My Dad Takes Care of Me

Stephanie and the Coyote

Sunshine

Ten, Nine, Eight

Songs

Free to Be ... a Family
  Another Cinderella
  The Day Dad Made Toast

Sing Your Sillies Out
  Daddy's Taking Us to the Zoo

Poems, Rhymes and Fingerplays

Where the Sidewalk Ends
  Helping

Objective 14
Jobs and Careers

Children will be able to name jobs or careers that men and women choose.

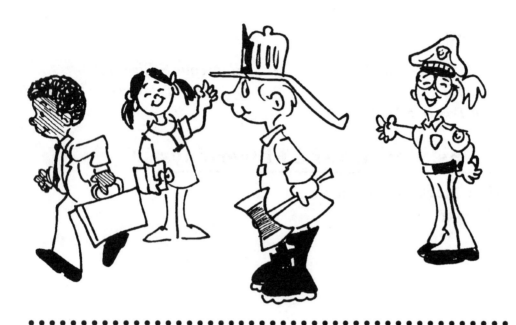

The purpose of this objective is to help children recognize and accept a variety of roles for men and women. Children should realize that all careers are open to either men or women.

If a person is capable of doing a job, he or she should be given the opportunity to do that job. Then he or she should perform the job to the best of his or her ability. No job is better than another, although some jobs require more training than others, some may pay more money and some are given more social respectability.

Every job is necessary and helps our community. Show how different jobs are important to the community. Discuss a variety of positions, such as sanitation worker, construction worker, fire fighter, doctor, secretary, etc.

Activities

Remembering Jobs

Remind the children of any previous classroom guests who talked about their careers. Show pictures of the guests to help children remember. Also remind children of any field trips and the people who worked where you visited.

Classroom Guests

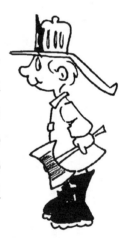

Invite several people to share information about their jobs with the children. Ask guests to bring props, so children can see some of their products or tools. Ask guests to tell the children if they had to go to school to learn how to do their job. Look for women and ethnic minorities in professional positions.

Look Closely

Select items from the classroom and help children see that they represent jobs of several people. For example:

Someone designed the puzzles; someone else may have cut the wood and painted the puzzles. Someone took pictures of the puzzles to put in a catalog (show children a catalog with puzzles in it). Someone mailed the catalog to the teacher. The mail carrier delivered it. Someone read the teacher's order, and someone else probably mailed the puzzle to the teacher.

Teaching

Tell the children that your job is to be their teacher. Explain briefly what your job involves. Give examples they will recognize, such as taking them outside or reading stories. Give examples they may not recognize, such as planning games, completing forms, etc.

Classified Ads

Show children the section of the newspaper that advertises work opportunities. Read a few examples to them. Explain that this is one way people find jobs.

Roleplay

Encourage children to act out each of the following jobs: doctor, teacher, hair stylist, construction worker, grocery store clerk, etc. Include careers that represent classroom

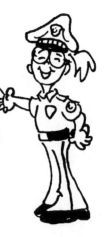

134

guests you have had and the family members of children in your classroom.

Traditional Learning Centers ....

Art

Display famous art works. Explain that artists created them. Posters and calendars are useful resources for famous pictures. Play music of famous composers and explain that creating music was their career.

Blocks

Hang pictures of many different types of structures, including castles. Add career block accessory dolls.

Housekeeping

Add uniforms representing many different kinds of careers.

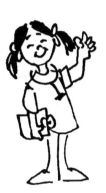

Manipulative

Add puzzles representing different careers.

Resources ●

More information on these resources can be found starting on p. 261.

Books

*Boys and Girls, Girls and
    Boys*
Curious George Takes a Job
Friday Night Is Papa's Night
Girls Can Be Anything
I Can Be a Truck Driver
Mommy Works on Dresses
Mothers Can Do Anything

My Daddy Is a Nurse
*My Mother Lost Her Job
    Today*
My Mother the Mail Carrier
Our Teacher's in a Wheelchair
Stories for Free Children
Tight Times

Songs

Baby Beluga
    Day O
Circle Around
    The Monster Song
Hug the Earth
    The Family Song
Singable Songs
    Baa Baa Black Sheep

Sing Your Sillies Out
    Fire Fighter
    Sanitation Engineer
When My Shoes Are Loose
    Bugs
Voyage for Dreamers
    Far Off Shore

Poems, Rhymes and Fingerplays

Free to Be ... a Family
    Something for Everyone

5.
Nutrition

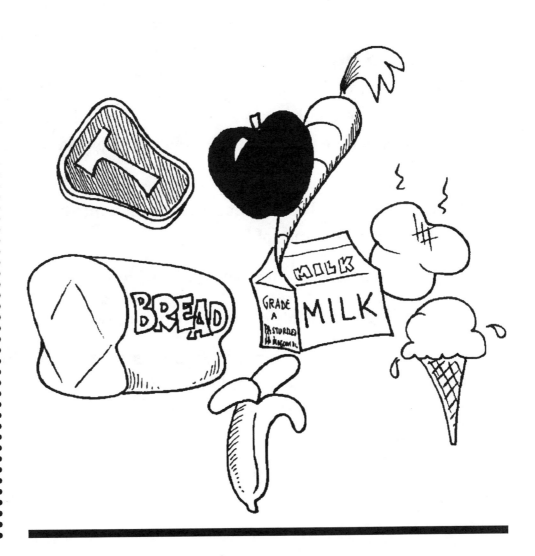

Nutrition

Young children can recognize food as the source of principal nutrients important for growth and health. Food helps meet body needs for proper growth and development. Children should eat a balanced diet that includes a variety of foods. Children can begin to recognize that some foods are not as nutritious as others.

Lifestyle Goals

Successful completion of this curriculum will put children on the road to developing the knowledge and motivation to:

- eat a daily diet that provides adequate nutrients for the maintenance of health;

- select foods representing a wide range of foodstuffs;

- balance calorie intake with energy needs;

- avoid dependence on food fads as the sole criterion for diet choices or meal planning.

Here We Go...Watch Me Grow!

Objective 15
Nutritious Snacks

Children will be able to identify nutritious snack foods.

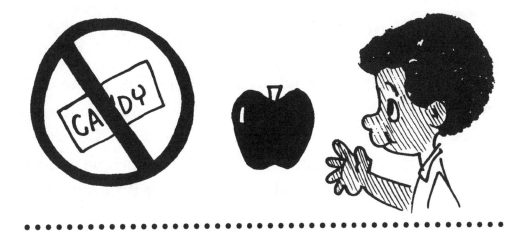

The purpose of this objective is to help children select nutritious snack foods when they are given a choice. Nutritious foods are those foods that help the body grow healthy and strong. Foods such as fresh fruits and vegetables, breads and milk are nutritious.

Foods that are high in fat and sugar, such as potato chips, candy, sodas and pastries, do not help the body as much. Foods high in salt should also be eaten in moderation.

Young children can easily recognize certain tastes, such as sweet and salty. These are acquired tastes that many children develop before three years of age.

Provide snack foods that taste good, yet are nutritious (low in sugar, salt and fat). Encourage children to select appropriate snacks. Explain the importance of establishing good eating habits.

Activities

Wind-Up Toy

Show a wind-up toy or music box to the children. Wind it up, and let children watch or listen to it slowly wind down. Look for other things that wind down. Let children act like the toy or music box. Discuss how people wind down or run down or get tired if they do not eat nutritious foods.

Sprouts

Let children sprout mung beans or alfalfa seeds. Cover seeds with water. Place a cover on the jar opening. A piece of screen or thin cloth or the lid with holes punched in it will work best. Soak the beans overnight. Drain the beans and put them in a warm, dark place. Rinse with cool water twice a day. Watch daily and record the changes on a class chart. Most sprouts will be ready to eat in five days.

Cooking with Children

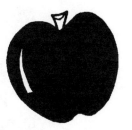

Fruit Salad: Let children prepare a fruit salad. Use a variety of fruits. You will need a knife, large bowl, large spoons, individual serving bowls or cups and individual spoons. Cut fresh fruits such as bananas, oranges, pineapples, apples, grapes and cantaloupes into bite-size pieces. (Remember that even grapes should be cut in half to reduce the chance of choking.) Sprinkle with coconut, or add a little orange juice if desired.

Sometimes children don't like foods mixed together. You can have a fruit bar with each of the fruits in a separate container. Children can decide for themselves whether to mix the fruit or eat it separately.

Carrot Salad: Let children wash carrots and then scrape them with a peeler. Let children use a grater and grate the carrots. Children can then stir the carrots into orange gelatin and make a congealed carrot salad.

Milkshake: Let children combine ice milk and orange juice in a blender to make an orange milkshake.

Where Does It Go?

Have pictures of nutritious foods and not-so-nutritious foods. Encourage children to sort the pictures into a box with a thumbs-up sign and the word *yes* on it for nutritious foods or a box with a thumbs-down sign and the word *no* on it for not-so-nutritious foods.

Mobiles

Let children make a nutritious snack mobile. This project may use real snacks such as carrot sticks or pictures of nutritious snacks.

Field Trips

Take a trip to a grocery store. Look for items that are nutritious, such as fruits, vegetables, bread and milk. If there is money available, purchase items to be used for snacks. For example: Shelled, unsalted sunflower or pumpkin seeds are nutritious and need no preparation. Nuts are not recommended because young children can easily choke on them.

Special Learning Centers

Grocery Store

Arrange boxes, cans, labels and pictures of nutritious foods. Later, add foods that are *not* nutritious. Provide a cash register and play money and paper bags and smocks for the store employees.

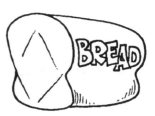

Traditional Learning Centers

Art

Hang pictures of food. Add stencils of food.

Blocks

Add various kinds of beans for children to haul in their play trucks.

Housekeeping

Add nutritious play food and food containers. Add washed apples for snacking.

Science

Provide tops of beets, carrots, turnips, sweet potatoes or parsnips and a large pie plate. Let children arrange the tops in the plate and add water to cover the bottom. Let them add small pebbles in between the tops. Children should add water and sunshine as needed.

Resources ·······················

More information on these resources can be found starting on p. 261.

Books

Bread and Jam for Frances
A Drop of Blood
Fat, Fat Calico Cat
Happy, Healthy Pooh Book

Let's Eat
Sweetie, a Sugar Coated
   Nightmare
The Sweet Touch

Songs

All of Us Will Shine
   Pearly White Waltz
And One and Two
   Raisins and Almonds
Baby Beluga
   All I Really Need
Learning Basic Skills
   Alice's Restaurant
One Light, One Sun
   Apples and Bananas

Singable Songs
   Five Little Frogs
   Peanut Butter Sandwich
Sing Your Sillies Out
   The Watermelon Song
When My Shoes Are Loose
   Do You Know
   Here Come the Bees
   I'm Just Hungry
   Worms

Poems, Rhymes and Fingerplays

Finger Frolics
   Ten Red Apples
   Ten Rosy Apples

Where the Sidewalk Ends
   Two Boxes

Objective 16
The Basic Four Food Groups

Children will be able to name foods found in each of the basic four food groups.

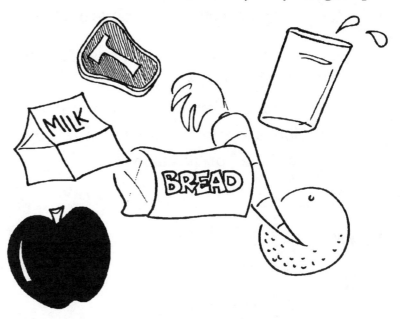

The purpose of this objective is to help children identify foods in the four food groups that contribute to healthy growth and development. Children should recognize the importance of eating a variety of foods.

The basic four food groups are meat and protein, fruits and vegetables, milk and cheese, and bread and cereal. These groups should be presented very simply. For example: The fruit and vegetable group includes all kinds of fruits and vegetables, including apples, carrots, green beans and bananas. The milk and cheese group includes all kinds of milk, yogurt, cheese, cottage cheese, milk shakes and ice cream. The protein and meat group includes all meats (chicken, hamburgers) fish, tofu and dried beans. The bread and cereal group includes rolls, buns, sliced bread, rice, tortillas, grits and all cereals.

It isn't appropriate to teach details such as the number of recommended servings in each food group. Tell children to eat a food from each group every day.

Foods found in the basic four food groups are nutritious. Foods such as cola drinks, candy and potato chips are high in fat and/or sugar or salt and are not-so-nutritious. These foods are not bad for you, but they don't help bodies grow as well as nutritious foods.

Activities

Where Does It Go?

Have play food or empty food containers to represent the basic four food groups. Let children sort play food or containers into four appropriate boxes. Each box  should have a picture and the words to show that food group. Example: *Milk and Cheese*—milk, chocolate milk, ice cream, yogurt.

Field Trips

Plan a trip to a grocery store. Look for foods from the four food groups.

Lotto

Make a lotto game with pictures of fruits and vegetables. Play the game with children.

Use pictures of meats to make a lotto game.

Make a milk and cheese lotto game.

Use pictures of breads and cereals to make a lotto game.

Menu Review

If your program serves lunch, read the lunch menu to children. Show pictures of each item on the menu. Choose one of the basic four food groups, and help children identify foods from that group that are on the menu. After discussing all of the groups separately, use the menu review time to categorize the foods being served that day.

Collages

Let children make a collage of the basic four food groups. Divide one large sheet of paper into four sections or use four different sheets. This can be a project for one day, or each food group can be covered on a separate day.

Let children make a group collage using pictures of a variety of foods.

Fruit Basket

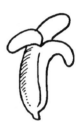

In a small group, show children a variety of fresh fruit. Let each child hold and smell the fruit. Talk about the name of each fruit. Let each child wash one piece of fruit and place it in a basket. Use the basket of fruit for a snack or part of a meal.

Vegetable Tray

In a small group, show children a variety of fresh vegetables. Let each child hold and smell the vegetables. Talk about the name of each vegetable. Let each child wash one piece and place it on a tray. Use the vegetable tray for a snack or part of a meal.

Bread Basket

In a small group, show children a variety of breads, such as muffins, English muffins, French bread, bagels, dinner rolls, etc. Also show children slices of whole-wheat and white bread. Explain that whole-wheat flour is better for their bodies. Let children wash their hands and taste different breads.

Traditional Learning Centers ....

Art

Provide cut fruits and vegetables for children to dip in paint and make prints on paper.

Housekeeping

Add play food and food containers representing the four food groups.

Manipulative

Add puzzles of the four food groups. Add games about the four food groups.

Resources ●●●●●●●●●●●●●●●●●●●●●●●●●●●●●●●●●●●●●

More information on these resources can be found starting on p. 261.

Books

Apple Pie and Onions

The Carrot Seed

Green Eggs and Ham

Look at You

Stone Soup

Ten Apples up on Top

Songs

Baby Beluga
  Biscuits in the Oven
  Day O
  Oats and Beans and Barley
Circle Around
  Vega Boogie
Everything Grows
  Everything Grows

Learning Basic Skills
  Alice's Restaurant
Singable Songs
  Aikendrum
  Apples and Bananas
Travellin' with Ella Jenkins
  Hukilau

Poems, Rhymes and Fingerplays

Finger Frolics
  Bread and Cereals
  Dairy Products
  Meat, Poultry and Seafood
  Vegetables and Fruits

Where the Sidewalk Ends
  Spaghetti

6.

Disease Prevention and Control

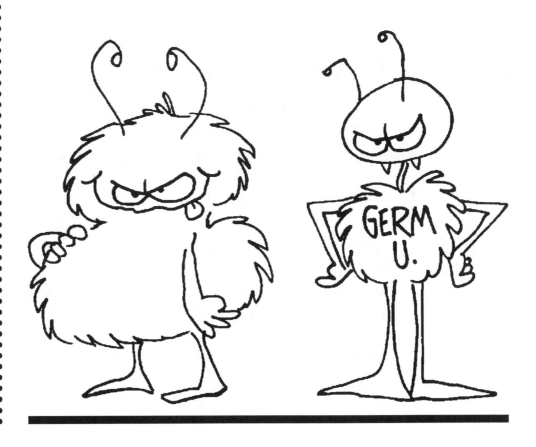

Disease Prevention and Control

In this unit, children study basic factors that contribute to the development of diseases and disorders. Preschool children can begin to understand what germs are and that germs are spread from person to person. It is not necessary to identify specific diseases that might frighten young children. The emphasis should be on personal cleanliness and hygiene.

Lifestyle Goals

Successful completion of this curriculum will put children on the road to achieving lifelong goals of:

- identifying and choosing lifestyle behaviors that promote well-being and minimize risk of disease and injury;

- maintaining immunizations of self and family at recommended levels of effectiveness;

- seeking preventive measures and professional assistance, such as examinations, at recommended intervals.

Objective 17
Wash Your Hands

*Children will be able to demonstrate
how to wash their hands.*

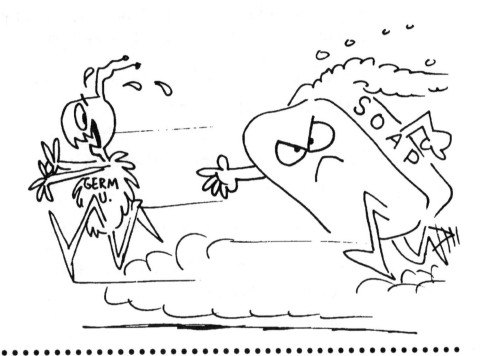

The purpose of this objective is to help children realize that even when their hands look clean, germs are still present and hands should be washed. Germs hide on the front and back of hands, between fingers and under nails. Stress careful washing in these areas during classroom demonstration and practice.

Teach children when they need to wash their hands, such as before eating or touching food, before setting the table and after using the toilet. Be sure that you serve as a role model by washing your hands at appropriate times, too.

Activities

Washing Hands

Demonstrate the proper way to wash hands. Correct technique includes washing around each hand (one hand moving over the other hand, both back and palm) and also scrubbing between fingers (interlock fingers and rub).

Show children that it is important to wash on both sides of the hands, between fingers and around and under fingernails. Let children practice washing their hands every day. In order to keep children interested in washing their hands, try these suggestions:

- Practice using different kinds of soap.

- Practice after holding an onion slice. Compare the smell to germs, because you cannot see either, but they are still there.

- Practice after you paint a germ on children's hands.

- Practice after rubbing lotion on children's hands, so they learn to rub all parts of their hands.

- Practice in a tub or a bowl full of water instead of the sink.

Bread Mold

This activity can be done for each child individually or as a class project. If it is a class project, use your own hands instead of a child's for the experiment. Explain the steps in the experiment. Ask children what they think will happen.

Wipe a clean hand or clean paintbrush on one slice of bread and a dirty hand or dirty paintbrush on another slice of bread. Put each slice in a separate jar and close the lid. Mark the jars as clean or dirty. Put both jars in a warm, dark place, such as a closet.

Check the progress to see which slice of bread produces molds most quickly. Record the progress with the children, and discuss the findings with them.

Problem Solving

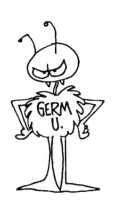

Ask children when it is important to wash their hands. Ask questions to encourage them to realize hand washing is needed after using the bathroom, before cooking, before handling eating utensils, before eating and after playing.

Puzzles

Help children make a dirty hands puzzle. Let them trace around their hand and then paint or color "dirt" on the hand. Then cut the paper hand into a few pieces and store in a container or envelope.

Shaving Cream

Let children use shaving cream to finger-paint on tables. The tables and children's hands will be clean at the end.

Daily Times

Arrange the schedule to include hand washing. Look at this as an opportunity for valuable learning time to practice positive health habits.

Doll Bath

Provide a time for children to give the dolls a bath. Encourage children to wash the dolls' hands, just as they wash their own hands.

Paint Wash

Use liquid soap and dry tempera to prepare finger paint. After children paint, let them wash their hands until all color is gone.

Look Close

Encourage children to use a magnifying glass to examine hands closely and search for specks of dirt.

Special Learning Centers

Water Play

Prepare a water center. (This is a traditional center for some classrooms.) If you do not have a water table, a wading pool, dishpan or any large container will work. Add water, liquid soap and eggbeaters for the area.

Traditional Learning Centers

Art

Add finger paint.

Blocks

Add a carwash for the vehicles. It can be a shoe box with holes cut in it and yarn attached for the water hose.

Housekeeping

Add water for washing dishes and clothes. Provide food such as peanut butter and crackers to prepare after washing hands.

Science

Add magnifying glasses to examine hands. Place dirt in a small container for children to put fingers in before examining their hands. Provide wet wipes for washing hands and re-examining them.

Resources ·····································

More information on these resources can be found starting on p. 261.

Books

Harry, the Dirty Dog
In the Forest

Tommy Takes a Bath
The Velveteen Rabbit

Songs

Baby Beluga
  Joshua Giraffe
Everything Grows
  Bathtime
Free to Be ... a Family
  Crowded Tub

Learning Basic Skills
  Keep the Germs Away
  Take a Bath
When My Shoes Are Loose
  Wash My Hands

Poems, Rhymes and Fingerplays

Finger Frolics
  Bath Time
  Caring for an Abrasion
  Dirty Hands
  Getting Dressed
  This Is the Way We...
  Washing Myself

Free to Be ... a Family
  Crowded Tub
Where the Sidewalk Ends
  The Dirtiest Man in the World
  Instructions
  Shadow Wash

Objective 18
Cover Your Mouth and Nose

Children will be able to explain why it is important to cover your mouth and/or nose before coughing or sneezing.

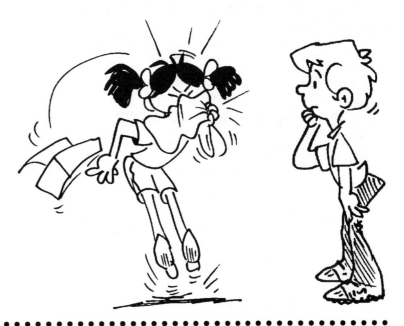

The purpose of this objective is to help children realize that germs cause diseases and that germs are spread from person to person in several ways.

Children can take individual responsibility to help control the spread of disease. Children learn best from real experiences; be sure to gently remind children to cover their mouths when they cough and cover their noses when they sneeze. Also, remind children to wash their hands after coughing or sneezing. Thank children who remember.

Activities

Spray It

Let children spray water on a piece of dark-colored paper. Explain that sneezes and coughs spray germs the same way water sprays on paper. Discuss the importance of covering your nose and/or mouth when sneezing or coughing.

Spray Paint

Prepare tempera paint and put it in spray bottles. Let the children spray paint a large sheet of paper. Stress the safety of spraying only the paper.

Warm Spray

Prepare warm soapy water for the children to use in a spray bottle to clean the tables in the room. Stress the safety of keeping the spray directed at the tables. Provide sponges and paper towels or old cleaning cloths. Explain that cleaning keeps germs away.

Demonstration to Assist in Nose Blowing

Young children often do not know how to blow their noses. Show children how to blow their noses, and explain

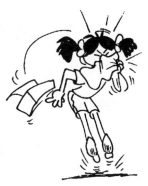

the process. Tell children that if they blow too hard, it can cause problems with their ears.

Use a variety of activities to demonstrate what blowing means. Select a few from these suggestions:

- Provide whistles for the children to blow when you point to them.

- Use straws for children to blow soapy water.

- Look around the building for things that blow, such as heat or air vents, fans, etc.

- Connect the hose of a vacuum cleaner to the exhaust end so that the air comes out. Have one child hold the hose so it is pointing up and have another child place a Ping-Pong ball in the stream of air.

Offer some activities to help children understand what sucking means and how it is different from blowing. Select a few from these suggestions:

- Provide straws to suck water or milk.

- Provide a vacuum cleaner for children to feel the suction and watch it clean or suck crumbs or dirt.

- Look around the building for things that have suction, such as an air conditioner intake vent.

- Provide a plunger for children to observe suction.

Someone Says

Use covering activities. Tell children to cover ears, toes, nose, eyes, knees, elbows, etc.

What Are Germs?

Read the dictionary definition to children. Tell children it is hard to understand things that can't be seen.

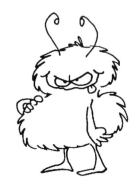

Little Made Big

Show children a microscope. Explain that it makes things look bigger than they are. Let children observe a blade of grass, a hair and a piece of thread. Explain that even with a microscope, we can't see some germs because the germs are so small.

Bubbles

Prepare bubble mixture by adding liquid detergent and sugar to water, or purchase bubble mixture. Use bubble blowers or any circular item with a hole in the center to let children practice blowing. Compare the bubbles to germs that move from place to place. After a bubble bursts, you can't see it either.

Traditional Learning Centers . . . .

Blocks

Add covered bridges. They can be shoe boxes with holes in the end turned upside down.

Housekeeping

Add blankets to cover the dolls. Add a tablecloth to cover the table.

Manipulative

Add puzzles and games with pictures of mouths, noses and hands.

Resources . . . .

More information on these resources can be found starting on p. 261.

Books

The Biggest Nose
The Giraffe Who Got in a Knot

I Wish I Was Sick, Too
Morris Has a Cold
The Velveteen Rabbit

Songs

Hug the Earth
  Skin
  Super Kids

Learning Basic Skills
  Cover Your Mouth

Poems, Rhymes and Fingerplays

Finger Frolics
  Blowing Bubbles
  I Godda Code

Where the Sidewalk Ends
  The Acrobats
  The Dirtiest Man in the World
  Sick

Objective 19
Medicines That Prevent Disease

Children will be able to explain that the purpose of immunizations is to protect us against some diseases.

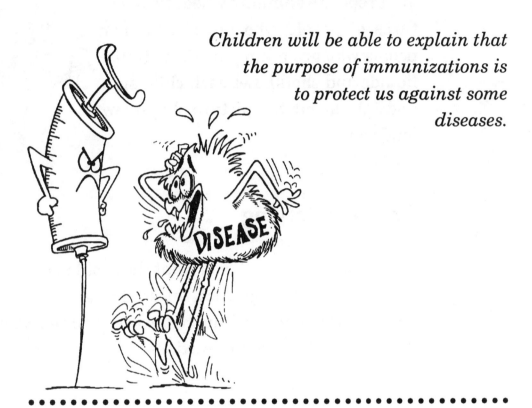

The purpose of this objective is to help children realize that sometimes they are given shots or medicine to make them well and sometimes the medicine or shots will keep them from getting sick.

Immunizations are medicines that prevent diseases. Some immunizations are shots and some are not. For example, drops or sugar cubes may be used for polio immunizations. Even if immunizations hurt, they are not as bad as being sick with the disease the medicine is used to prevent. However, not all illnesses are preventable.

Activities

Spinning Wheel

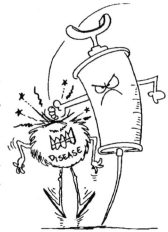

Prepare a spinning wheel with pictures of people who are sick and/or people who are taking medicine (pills, liquids and shots). Let each child spin and talk about the picture the arrow lands on.

Problem Solving

Ask children to tell you what they could do to keep from getting too tired, angry, hot, thirsty, hungry or cold. Ask one question at a time. Explain that to keep from getting certain illnesses we take immunizations.

Brainstorming

List ways we prevent illness. Encourage ideas such as wearing warm clothes, covering sneezes and coughs, immunizations, exercise, good nutrition, etc.

Language Experience Story

Encourage children to tell stories about when they got immunizations. They may remember a time they got shots.

Write down everything they say. Read it back to them after they are finished.

It's a Rule

Show children a copy of daycare regulations or school rules. Explain that just like classroom rules, there are rules for schools and all daycare centers. Read to children *briefly* the rule about immunizations. Explain that the reason for the rule is to keep everyone healthy.

Special Learning Centers

Water Play

Provide a container of water and syringes *without* needles for children to play with. Talk with children about how the syringe works. Tell children that instead of water, immunizations contain medicine to help them stay well.

Traditional Learning Centers

Art

Add a syringe (without a needle) to the paint area.

Blocks

Provide a container for all blocks to go into if they have rough edges. Sand the blocks that need it and return them to the block center. Explain that sanding helps prevent any injury due to splinters, just as immunizations prevent certain diseases.

Housekeeping

Place bandages on the dolls' arms, and explain that the dolls had their immunizations.

Manipulative

Add doctor puzzles and games.

Resources
• •

More information on these resources can be found starting on p. 261.

Books

My Doctor
No Measles, No Mumps for
  Me

Songs

Learning Basic Skills
  Keep the Germs Away

Poems, Rhymes and Fingerplays

Where the Sidewalk Ends
  Oh Have You Heard

Objective 20
Sharing Food and Drinks

Children will be able to explain the healthy way to share food and drinks.

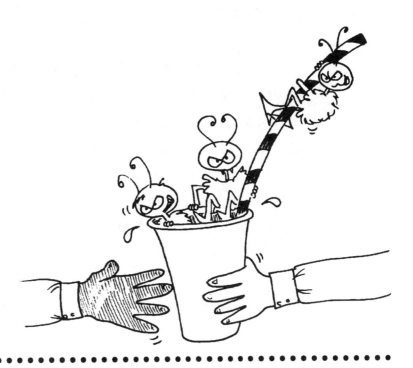

The purpose of this objective is to show how sharing items such as drinking glasses can spread germs. Germs can live on inanimate (non-living) objects, such as food and eating utensils. Some of these germs can cause diseases. Young children share a variety of items ranging from toys to sandwiches.

While sharing is encouraged, there are *healthy* ways to share food. If two children want to share a sandwich, they should cut it in half before either of them takes a bite. If sharing a beverage, they should pour it into separate glasses before either tastes it.

Activities

Sharing

Talk about what sharing means. Explain that healthy sharing means sharing food and drink before we eat or drink any. Hold up a spoon, and tell children they should not share their spoons with others. Hold up a fork, and ask if they should share their forks. Compare the fork to the spoon. Hold up a cup, and ask if they should share it. Also hold up some toys that would be acceptable to share.

Discovery Box

Place a spoon, fork, napkin, plate, straw, car, block, crayon, book or other objects into the Discovery Box. Encourage children to feel the item and guess if it is something they should or should not share with others.

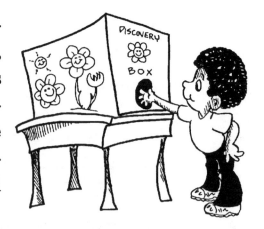

If the answer is to share, ask *how* they can share it. This will help avoid misunderstanding. For example, children might be willing to let someone use a clean spoon because

Here We Go...Watch Me Grow!

they can get another spoon from the teacher. Children might be willing to share a cookie (wrapped in plastic) if they break the cookie in half before either person takes a bite.

Someone Says

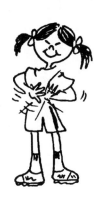

Use commands with the word *before*. For example: "Mieko says, 'Stand up *before* you jump up and down'"; "April says, 'Stretch up high *before* you lie down'"; "Carlos says, 'Clap your hands *before* you stand up.'"

Problem Solving

Have eating utensils and a variety of food in a picnic basket. Hold up one item, and ask children to tell you how they could share it in a healthy way. Can it be cut? Are there two of the same items? Can it be shared using a spoon to divide it, if no one has eaten with the spoon? Can it be poured into separate cups? Explore the options.

Classroom Guest

Invite a police officer to show children how fingerprints are discovered on evidence. Ask the officer to use the children's prints to demonstrate. Explain that just as fingerprints are left on objects children touch, germs are left on foods children touch or put in their mouths.

Where Does It Go?

Collect a variety of items that are appropriate to share (cars, crayons, blocks) and some that are unhealthy to share (spoon, straw, napkin, plate). Ask children to sort the items into a share basket and a not-to-share basket.

Sharing Snack

At snack time explain that some of the children will get a snack and share it with others. After all the children wash their hands, give half of them a healthy drink and snack.

Tell children to pour half of their drink into another cup to share *before* they take a drink. Since young children may not understand *half,* you can draw a line on the empty cup and tell children to fill it to that line.

There may be spills. Have sponges or paper towels available for children to use to clean up spills. Assure children that they will receive more to drink, and encourage them to try again.

Ask children to share the snack. Tell them to cut the snack food in half *before* they take a bite. Or if they have more than one piece of the snack food, they can offer to let another child take one piece. Children should touch only the piece they take. During the next snack time, let the other children share in the same way.

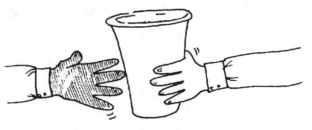

Traditional Learning Centers

Housekeeping

Add a pitcher of drinking water and paper cups for the children to share. Assist children to share in a healthy way. Add whole-wheat, low-salt crackers for snack or learning center time. Assist children in healthy sharing.

Resources

More information on these resources can be found starting on p. 261.

Books

Bread and Jam for Frances   *Gooseberries to Oranges*
Everybody Takes Turns   *Stone Soup*

Songs

And One and Two   *Singable Songs*
   Sharing   *The Sharing Song*

Poems, Rhymes and Fingerplays

Where the Sidewalk Ends
   My Stew

7.

Safety and First Aid

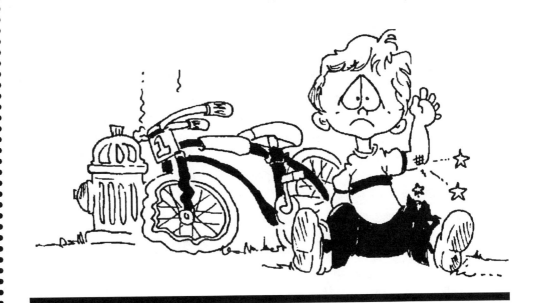

Safety and First Aid

In this unit, children are introduced to methods for identifying and eliminating hazardous conditions or situations. Children should understand rules and procedures for safe living in the home, school and community. This unit is designed to help prevent accidents and teach basic first aid and emergency care.

Lifestyle Goals

Successful completion of this curriculum will put children on the road to achieving lifelong goals of:

- taking steps to correct hazardous conditions when possible;

- following rules and procedures recommended for safe living;

- avoiding unnecessary risk-taking behavior;

- applying correct emergency treatment when appropriate;

- being able to contact emergency sources of help.

Objective 21
Traffic Signs and Signals

Children will be able to describe the meaning of traffic signs and signals.

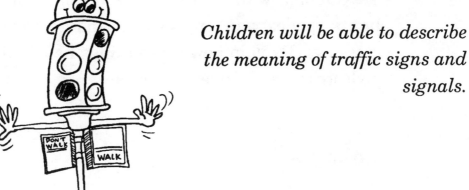

The purpose of this objective is to help children become more responsible for their own safety. Include the following signs and signals: red, yellow and green lights; walk/don't walk signals; pedestrian crossing sign; stop sign; and railroad sign.

Drivers, bicyclists and pedestrians must obey traffic rules and signs. Traffic rules and signs provide for the safety of everyone. Actual experiences, such as field trips to low-traffic areas, will help children observe examples of safety signs and signals and discuss their importance.

Activities ······························

Walks

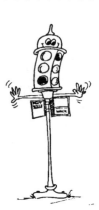

Go for a walk. Look for traffic signs and lights, pedestrian crosswalks and railroad crossings. Explain how these things help both pedestrians and drivers to be safe.

Collages

Let children make a red and green collage. The colors can be divided or mixed together. Have children cut and tear pieces of paper of different textures to place on the background paper.

Lotto

Use a variety of traffic signs to make a lotto game. Play traffic sign lotto.

Spinning Wheel

Make a spinning wheel with pictures of traffic signs. Encourage each child to spin the arrow and talk about the picture the arrow lands on.

Special Learning Centers

Traffic Path

Set up a traffic path either inside or outside the classroom. Arrange streets with signs for the children to walk or ride tricycles on. Use actual street names from the children's neighborhoods to name the streets.

Colorful Water

Provide several clear plastic containers of water and red and green food color. Let children experiment.

Water Play

Add red food coloring to the water in the play area.

Traditional Learning Centers

Art

Display pictures of safety signs.

Blocks

Include block accessory safety signs.

Manipulative

Add puzzles with pictures of safety signs.

Resources •••

More information on these resources can be found starting on p. 261.

Books

Automobiles for Mice
Clifford, the Small Red Puppy
CROSS

Make Way for Ducklings
When I Cross the Street

Songs

And One and Two
   I'm Going to School Today
Baby Beluga
   Biscuits in the Oven
Learning Basic Skills
   Safe Way
   Stop, Look and Listen

Singable Songs
   Bumping up and Down
Sing Your Sillies Out
   Riding in My Car
   Transportation
Voyage for Dreamers
   Shadow of a Life

Poems, Rhymes and Fingerplays

Finger Frolics
   At the Curb
   Corner
   Look Both Ways
   Traffic Lights

Where the Sidewalk Ends
   Traffic Light

Objective 22
Community Safety Helpers

Children will be able to describe the roles of community safety helpers.

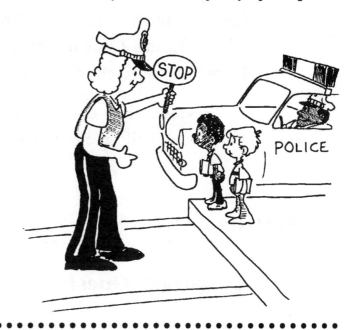

The purpose of this objective is to help children become familiar with the roles and responsibilities of community safety personnel and to understand that everyone has a responsibility for community safety.

Community safety personnel may include police officers, fire fighters, school crossing guards and paramedics. Emphasize that both men and women can be community safety personnel. Avoid using words such as *policeman* and *fireman*, which suggest that these jobs are for men only. Use *police officer* and *fire fighter*.

Even though safety personnel have different roles, they all work together for the good of the entire community. Encourage children to explore ways they can improve safety.

You may also wish to teach children how to call for help. If your area has a 911 emergency number, teach children to use 911. Remember, children must learn to use both rotary-dial and push-button telephones. Be sure children know what a *9* and a *1* look like on the phone. If your area does not have 911, teach children to dial *0* for operator.

Review what children should say in an emergency. Have each child recite his or her name and address.

Activities ....

Classroom Guests

Invite one or more community safety helpers to visit (police officer, fire fighter, ambulance driver, bus driver or crossing guard). Be prepared for a variety of responses from children, depending on their personal experiences with safety personnel.

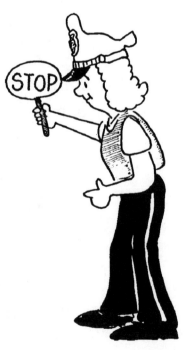

Roleplay

Provide safety personnel uniforms, and let children try on different ones. Encourage children to act like they are doing the job of a worker who would wear that uniform. Videotape the event, and play the safety show for the children to enjoy.

Problem Solving

Display pictures, puppets or dolls of a police officer, fire fighter, ambulance attendant, crossing guard and any other community safety helper. Be sure to have women and minorities represented.

Present the following situations. Ask children which safety worker would come to help. Create other situations to go along with the pictures or figures of safety workers you have displayed.

- There is a fire at your school.

- Someone breaks into your house and steals toys.

- A woman is hit by a car.

- There is a fire at your home.

- A car had a wreck.

- Children need help crossing the street.

- There is a fire at the grocery store.

- Someone is hurting another person.

- You are outside playing, and you find a gun in the bushes.

Field Trips

Visit any place where community safety personnel work, such as the fire station or police department.

911/0

Show children real telephones, some with touch buttons and others with rotary dials. Show as many varieties of telephones as possible. Explain that people use telephones to call community safety helpers when they need help.

Show children a telephone book. Explain that the fire department and the police department each have separate telephone numbers, just like your home telephone number is different from your friend's telephone number. Look up some numbers to show the children.

Explain that when people really need help fast, it is called an *emergency*. In emergencies, people can call police, fire or ambulance workers by dialing the numbers *911* or *0*. Tell children that since the telephones are not plugged in during class, if you dial a number it will not ring anywhere.

Roleplay for them, calling *911* or *0* (whichever is appropriate for your community). Then let children report a fire, a sick person and someone breaking into their house.

Tell children that if there is a fire, calling from another house is safer.

Let children dial *911* or *0* and report an emergency on the real telephone (unplugged). ***Help children understand that they should not call 911 or 0 unless it is an emergency.*** If you have enhanced-911 in your area, explain that to the children.

Special Learning Centers

Safety Offices

Set up areas of the room or playground to serve as offices for each of the following: police officer, fire fighter, ambulance driver, bus driver, crossing guard. Include props to encourage roleplay. *Do not* include weapons.

Traditional Learning Centers

Blocks

Add safety vehicles such as police cars, ambulances and fire trucks. Add safety helper dolls.

Housekeeping

Add safety helper uniforms to the dress-up clothes.

Manipulative

Add puzzles and games with pictures of safety helpers.

Resources ....

More information on these resources can be found starting on p. 261.

Books

The Trouble with Mom
When I Cross the Street

When There Is a Fire, Go
   Outside

Songs

Free to Be ... a Family
   On My Pond

Sing Your Sillies Out
   Fire Fighter
   Sanitation Engineer

Poems, Rhymes and Fingerplays

(Note: The following fingerplays would be appropriate to use if the words fire fighter *are substituted for* fireman *and* police officer *for* policeman. *The word* he *should sometimes be replaced by* she.)

Finger Frolics
   The Crossing Guard
   The Fireman

   Mr. Policeman
   Traffic Policeman

Objective 23
Safety Rules

Children will be able to explain the purpose of school and home safety rules.

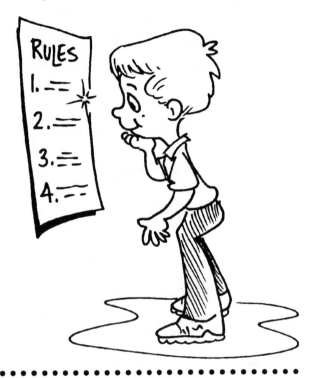

The purpose of this objective is to help children learn safety rules and understand reasons for having rules.

Since young children have difficulty understanding and remembering rules, the teacher's role is to provide a safe environment with close supervision. Teachers can help children learn rules by gently reminding children during real situations. Modeling and encouragement are essential.

You may include rules for the classroom, playground, halls, buses or emergency drills. Choose only those rules which are most important to the child's safety and well-being. Three-year-old children, and some four- and five-year-old children, do not usually understand or remember rules.

Guidance reasons that are specific to a real situation and are practiced often are more likely to be remembered. You may ask the children to discuss similar rules that they have at home. Take the children through the steps of identifying, understanding and practicing/following rules.

Activities ••••••••••••••••••••••••••••••••••••••

Safety Rules

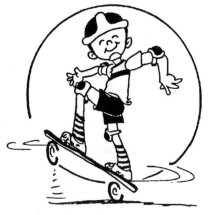

Review and/or establish school safety rules. Encourage children to help you establish the rules. Write and illustrate the rules. Use positive instead of negative words. For example: Walk in the hall-ways, rather than do not run in the hall.

Signal

Establish an emergency signal, such as flashing the lights, ringing a bell, etc. Teach it to children and practice using it. Do not use it to get the children's attention daily. If you are located in a public building with alarms, familiarize the children with the sound to avoid fear or confusion in a true emergency.

Someone Says

Someone Says gives children practice in following directions. After one-step commands have been accomplished, work on two, three and four steps given at once. Examples: (1) Hop on one foot. (2) Hop on one foot and touch your nose. (3) Touch your head, close your eyes, and wave your hand.

Emergency Drills

Practice emergency procedures with children. Do practices at times other than when the entire building is having a drill (fire, tornado, earthquake, etc.). Demonstrate and explain what you want children to do and why.

Exits

With the children, draw a floor plan of the classroom and/or building. Draw places where the exits (doors and windows) are. Let the children find the word EXIT if it is posted.

Walks

Walk through the building or a nearby building and look for EXIT signs.

Special Learning Centers ....

The Safety Area

Arrange an area that includes safety items such as the emergency route (fire escape plan), safety belts, eye protection goggles, hard hats, etc. Encourage children to explore and discuss the items.

Traditional Learning Centers ....

Art

Label where each item is to be returned. Post any rules for the art center.

Blocks

Label where each item is to be returned. Post any rules for the block center.

Housekeeping

Label where each item is to be returned. Post any rules for the housekeeping center.

Manipulative

Label where each item is to be returned. Post any rules for the manipulative center.

Science

Label where each item is to be returned. Post any rules for the science center.

Resources •

More information on these resources can be found starting on p. 261.

Books

Happy, Healthy Pooh Book
Look at You
Mr. Grumpy's Outing

Play It Safe
Strangers
When I Cross the Street

Songs

And One and Two
  I'm Going to School Today
Learning Basic Skills
  Keep the Germs Away
  Safe Way
  Stop, Look and Listen

When My Shoes Are Loose
  Legs, Slow Down
  Pick It Up
  Wash My Hands

<u>Poems, Rhymes and Fingerplays</u>

Where the Sidewalk Ends
   My Rules

Objective 24
What to Put in Your Mouth

Children will be able to identify various items that are safe (or dangerous) to put in the mouth.

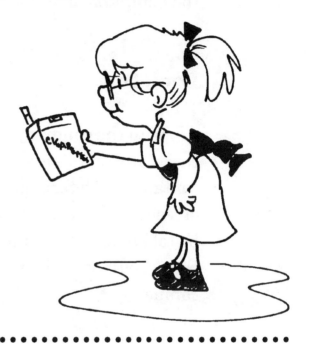

The purpose of this objective is to help children understand that they should put only safe food items in their mouths. Many substances may look like food and even smell or taste good, but they might be poisonous and can make a child very sick.

Discuss nonfood items that are commonly put into mouths. Examples should include tobacco products. Another danger of putting nonfood items in the mouth is choking. Children should never put toys, coins, pins or other objects in their mouths.

Activities •

Poisons

Tell children that there is a book called a dictionary. Show them one and explain what it is. Then read to them the definition of *poison*.

Look Out

With the children, look in the room or building to see if there are containers that may contain poisons. When a container is determined to be hazardous, put a skull and crossbones picture or an *X* on it. *Important:* Children should be told that if they find any poisonous items or chemicals, they should give them to an adult to be stored in a locked cabinet.

Walks

Go for a walk and watch animals, birds and insects eat. Explain that people do not necessarily eat the same things that animals eat. Ask children, "What things do animals eat that also look like food to us?"

To Eat or Not

Collect pictures of food and nonfood items, and place them in a container. Have children select a picture. If the picture is of food, the child throws a bean bag into a bucket with a picture of food on it. If the picture is not food, the child throws the bean bag into a different bucket. For the nonfood pictures, be sure to have pictures of substances that may be poisonous (such as cleaning agents or plants) as well as pictures of toys or other objects that might create choking hazards.

Field Trips

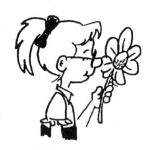

Visit a nursery or flower shop. Ask the workers to point out plants that are poisonous. (Call before going to be sure the staff knows which plants are poisonous.) You may want to contact a nearby children's hospital or poison control center and get a poster with pictures of poisonous plants, so you can identify them yourself.

Where Does It Go?

Place play food and toys into a basket. Make another container with a mouth. This may be a coffee can with the lid cut and painted like lips. Children select an item from the basket. The play food goes into the container with the mouth. The toys go into a different container.

Problem Solving

Ask children what they could do if they wanted to eat a berry but didn't know if it was poisonous. Be sure to explain that things that are poisonous can make you very sick or even cause death.

Tobacco

Show the children chewing tobacco, cigarettes, pipes and cigars. Let children touch them and talk about them. Explain that children should *not* put these things in their mouths. Tell children it is not healthy to use any of these products.

Some children may be concerned because a parent smokes. Explain that smoking is a habit and that it is hard not to smoke, once you start. Emphasize that smokers are not *bad,* but the smoke from their cigarettes can hurt their bodies and your body.

Traditional Learning Centers ·······················

Art

Add a scrapbox for small pieces of paper, bottle caps, cotton balls, etc., for children to use in collages.

Add bird feeder materials, and let children create different types. Pine cones can be stuffed with peanut butter and cornmeal and attached to a string for hanging. Ears of corn can be tied with a string and hung in a tree.

Blocks

Add beans or small rocks for hauling in trucks.

Housekeeping

Add imaginative (pretend) foods such as pine cones and rocks. Explain that these things are not to be put into the mouth. Supervise closely.

Science

Prepare a string or cardboard ring 1-1/2 inches in diameter. Let children use it to measure infant toys. Have the toys sorted into safe and unsafe categories. All toys smaller than 1-1/2 inches in diameter are unsafe for infants. *Caution:* Before using this activity, be sure all the children can safely participate without placing items in their mouths.

Resources ●●

More information on these resources can be found starting on p. 261.

Books

Blue Bug to the Rescue   *Play It Safe*
I Know an Old Lady

Songs

When My Shoes Are Loose
   Bugs
   Worms

Poems, Rhymes and Fingerplays

Finger Frolics   *Where the Sidewalk Ends*
   Five Little Sparrows   *Alice*
   Ten Little Pigeons   *Boa Constrictor*
                           Early Bird
                           If the World Was Crazy
                           Melinda Mae
                           Recipe for a Hippopotamus
                              Sandwich
                           Sky Seasoning

Objective 25
Never Play with Weapons

Children will be able to explain what to do if they find a weapon.

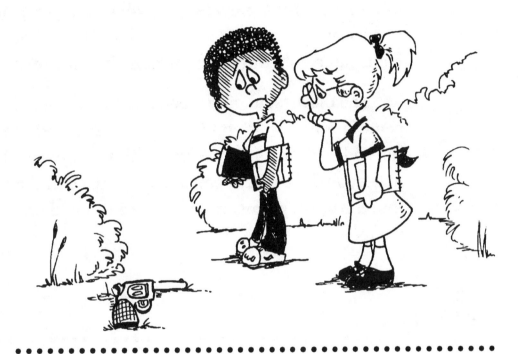

The purpose of this objective is to help children prevent accidental injury from guns, knives, or bows and arrows. Some adults keep guns in their homes. Children may not recognize the difference between a real weapon and a toy. They must learn that *all* guns should be considered *real* and that they are potentially loaded.

Teach children *never* to pick up a gun, even if they think it is a toy or unloaded. Tell children *never* to point a gun, even a toy, at another person or at themselves. If another child or someone other than a parent picks up a gun, children should tell that person to put the gun down. If he or she does not, the child should *leave immediately and tell a responsible adult.*

Knives can also be dangerous weapons. Teach children that knives are very sharp and can be dangerous. Tell children they should *never* play with kitchen knives, pocket knives or hunting knives. They should *never* even pretend to cut someone with a knife. Accidents can happen, and a child can easily hurt him- or herself or someone else.

The discussion of weapons can be a sensitive issue in some families. Help children understand that the *weapon* is not bad. Neither is the person (such as the parent) who owns a weapon. However, weapons can be used in the wrong way and can be very dangerous. Children should *never* play with weapons.

Activities

Weapon

Tell children that a weapon is anything used to fight with someone or hurt someone. Ask them if they can give examples. If they can't, then give them some examples, such as guns, rifles, knives, etc.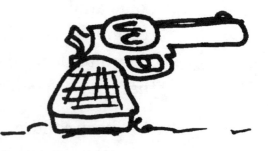

Circle Share

Ask children to tell you about a time they saw someone hold or use a weapon. The time can be real or on a television show. Ask what happened to the victim (explain *victim*). Help children see that weapons hurt people and sometimes kill them. Remind children that anything they saw on a television show was not real and those people are okay.

Problem Solving

Ask children why they think people fight with weapons.

Ask children to think of ways to solve problems without fighting with weapons.

Ask children what they think they should do if they find a gun (or knife or other weapon). Help them understand that they should *not* pick it up or touch it, even if they think it may be a toy.

Ban Weapons

In your classroom, ban the use of all weapons, even imaginary ones. Explain that weapons can hurt people and you want the classroom to be a safe place for children.

Traditional Learning Centers

All Centers

Place pictures of weapons. Hide some under the blocks and under puzzle pieces. Tell children to come and get you as soon as they see one and not to touch any of them.

Art

Add spray bottles with paint. Explain that bullets come out of a gun and hit things or people just as the paint comes out of the bottle and hits the paper. The difference is that the paint does not hurt the paper. The bullet will hurt a person.

Resources

More information on these resources can be found starting on p. 261.

Books

A Bargain for Frances
Drummer Hoff
The Hating Book
The Hunter and the Animals
Let's Be Enemies
Mr. Grumpy's Motor Car
Play with Me

The Quarreling Book
Something Is Wrong at My House
The Story of Ferdinand
Two Good Friends
Where the Wild Things Are

Songs

Free to Be ... a Family
   The Turn of the Tide
Peace Is the World Smiling
   If I Had a Hammer
   We Love Our Home
   Whale Gulch Rap

Teaching Peace
   Teaching Peace
Voyage for Dreamers
   Moon Spirit
When My Shoes Are Loose
   Bugs
   Here Come the Bees

Poems, Rhymes and Fingerplays

Where the Sidewalk Ends
   Hug O'War

Objective 26
Using Seat Belts and Car Seats

Children will be able to demonstrate proper use of seat belts and/or car safety seats.

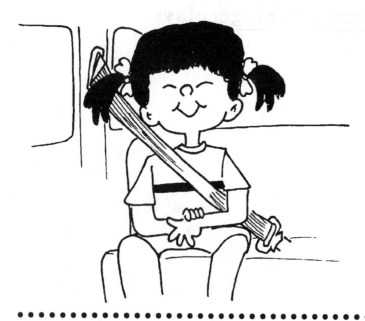

• •

The purpose of this objective is to teach the importance of using a seat belt *every time* you are in a vehicle. Everyone in the vehicle should use a seat belt.

Automobile accidents are one of the greatest causes of accidental injury and death for both young children and adults. Buckling a seat belt and keeping young children in car seats are the most important things anyone can do to prevent injury. Children can encourage parents to wear seat belts and can teach younger children to buckle up.

Here We Go...Watch Me Grow!

Remember that seat belts can only work if they are used properly.

Find out the law for the use of car seats and seat belts in your state. Many preschoolers will still be using a car seat.

Activities

Circle Share

Invite children to tell about any car accidents they have seen or have experienced. Be sensitive to any serious accidents.

Field Trips

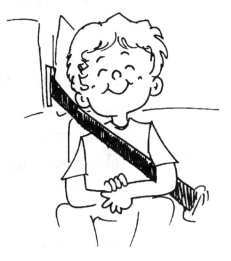

Take a few children at a time on a field trip to the parking lot to get into a vehicle with seat belts. Let children practice putting seat belts on in the front seat and in the back seat. Let children try several different cars with different seat belts if available.

Construct Cars

As a group, use cardboard boxes to make cars and trucks. Be sure that each car has a seat belt that children can operate alone. You may want to look in discount stores or secondhand stores for old belts (adult size) that can be laced through holes in the box car.

Belt Buckle

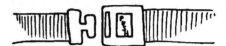

Provide many different seat belts that fasten a variety of ways. Encourage children to try on the different belts and learn to fasten them. You may be able to borrow samples of seat belts from your local traffic safety or police department.

Car Seats

Provide as many car seats (infant and toddler) as possible for the children to see. Explain that these seats keep young children and babies safe, just as seat belts keep older children and adults safe. Let children buckle up the classroom dolls or stuffed animals.

Sudden Stop

Play music for the children to move to. When the music stops, tell children to stop and hold the same position until the music begins again. Try fast and slow music. Tell children that when a car is moving and stops, seat belts help hold us in our seats. Without seat belts, we might fall or lean forward, etc.

Traditional Learning Centers

Art

Hang colorful belts in the art area.

Blocks

Add yarn seat belts to any vehicle in the block area.

Housekeeping

Add belts to the dress-up area. Add car seats for the dolls.

Science

Add seat belts that fasten in different ways for children to explore. Automobile salvage businesses may provide seat belts for you.

Manipulative

Add puzzles and games with pictures of vehicles.

Resources ....

More information on these resources can be found starting on p. 261.

Books

Automobiles for Mice
Play It Safe

Safe Sally Seatbelt and the
  Magic Click
When I Ride in a Car

Songs

Learning Basic Skills
  Buckle Your Seat Belt

Sing your Sillies Out
  Wheels

Objective 27
In Case of Fire

Children will be able to demonstrate appropriate action in case of fire.

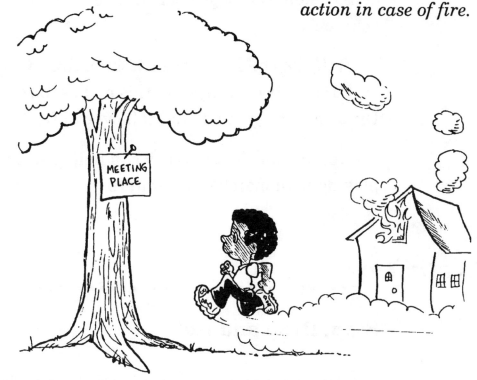

The purpose of this objective is to help children prevent unnecessary injury from fire. There are three main concepts to teach children:

1. In case of a house or school fire: The most important action is to *get out safely*. Do not try to put out the fire yourself. Families should have an evacuation plan for the home, just as schools do. This plan must specify a meeting place that is a safe distance from the building. If children go to the meeting place, then their family or teacher will know they are safe and will not continue to look for them.

Children should know these evacuation plans and should practice them.

2. If the child sees a fire: Go to the nearest adult and tell him or her to get people out (if necessary) and/or call the fire department. Do *not* go near the fire or try to put out the fire yourself.

3. If the child's clothes catch on fire: **Stop, drop and roll**. Do not try to run, since this makes the fire burn faster. Drop onto the ground, and roll over until the fire is out.

Teach children that they can help prevent fires by not playing with matches or lighters.

Activities ....

Stop, Drop and Roll

Explain that if children's clothes are on fire, they need to **stop, drop and roll** to put out the fire. Let children practice this.

Practice

Practice fire drills. Time the drill and let children know if they were fast enough. Let children discuss the fire drills.

Fire Spreads

Let children use an eyedropper to drop water on a paper towel or tissue. Encourage them to watch how the water spot gets bigger—even though more water is not added. Explain that fire is like that. It spreads over an area.

Burning House

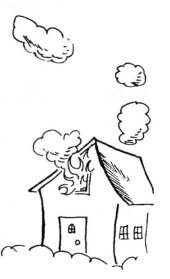

Make a doll house for small dolls. Put the dolls in the house in different places. Put a red construction paper flame somewhere on or in the house. Ask children what they think each person in the house should do. Remind children about not running, but getting out of the building in case of a fire.

Surveys

Ask children to survey their family members and find out what to do in case of fire at home. Every family member should know one place *away from the house* where the family will meet in case of fire. This will help fire fighters know if everyone has left the house safely.

Play Things

Place matches, a lighter and toys in a container. Pull out objects one at a time, and ask if each is a toy. If yes, ask how children could play with it. When you pull out matches or the lighter, see if children know what they are. Tell children these are *not* toys. **Note: Do not leave matches and lighters within the reach of children.**

Traditional Learning Centers

Blocks

Add fire trucks to the block area.

Housekeeping

Add a small empty fire extinguisher. Remove the pull pin first as a safety precaution. Add temporary fire detectors to the housekeeping area and explain how they work.

Manipulative

Add puzzles and games with pictures of fire, fire fighters, firetrucks or smoke. Add fire fighter puppets.

Resources . . . .

More information on these resources can be found starting on p. 261.

Books

Fire! Fire! Said Mrs. McGuire

Grumbel, the Fire-Breathing
 Dragon

When There Is a Fire, Go
 Outside

Songs

Learning Basic Skills
 Safe Way

Sing Your Sillies Out
 Fire Fighter

8.

Consumer Health

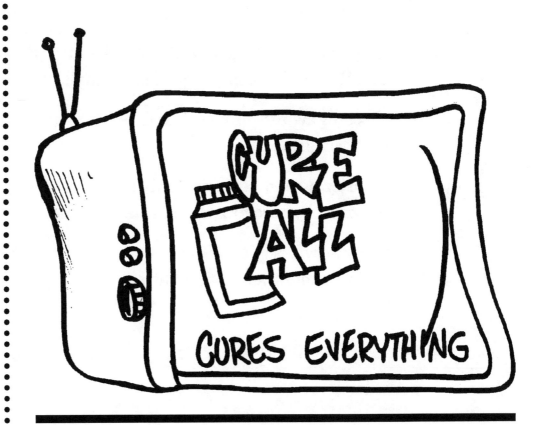

Consumer Health

This unit introduces children to the forces of advertising that influence our selection of health information, products and services as well as reasons for those selections. Young children can recognize commercials that motivate the sale and purchase of health-related products and services.

Lifestyle goals

Successful completion of this curriculum will put children on the road to achieving lifelong goals of:

- choosing health products and services on the basis of valid criteria;

- identifying and accepting only that health information provided by recognized health authorities;

- using services of qualified health advisors to maintain and promote their own health.

What Are Commercials?

Children will be able to explain that the purpose of advertisements is to sell products.

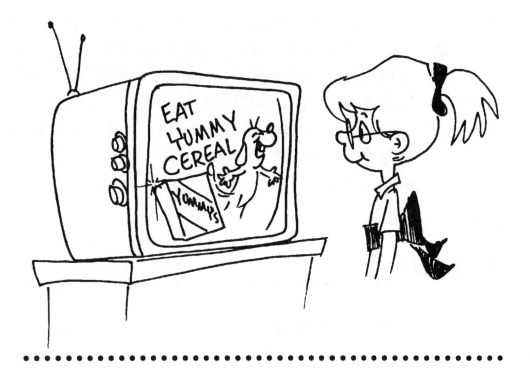

The purpose of this objective is to teach children that advertisements are made to sell a product, service or idea—such as the Say No to Drugs campaign. These ideas, products or services may or may not be necessary or even good for us.

One difficulty for preschool age children is that they may not be able to distinguish between commercials and the actual program. For example, famous characters are portrayed not only in cartoon programs, but often in advertisements for cereal products as well.

A second difficulty is that children generally believe everything that an adult tells them. The exception to this is the concept of *good guys* and *bad guys*. If children perceive an adult as a *bad guy,* they may not believe the adult. People in advertisements are neither good nor bad. They are simply trying to sell their products.

Explore different ways people sell products. Advertisements during Saturday morning cartoons specifically target children. Advertisements for the 1-900-telephone numbers also target children. Children may not realize that these telephone calls cost money and that the stories they may hear on the telephone are not any better than the stories people they know read to them.

Activities ●●●

Brainstorming

Ask, "Why are there commercials?" It may be necessary to watch a few commercials first and help all children understand what a commercial is. Explain that commercials are made to get you to buy something. They also help us find things we want to buy.

Brainstorm things that cannot be bought. Examples are friends, family members and feelings. Explain that some advertisements for churches, clubs, etc., promote an idea, not a product.

Advertisement Project

Encourage children to make a product. This can be an individual or group project. When the product is finished, ask children to tell you about it. Ask about color, texture, shape and use.

Let children decide how the product could be advertised and help them as needed. Depending on the availability of equipment, give children choices of talking on a tape player (radio), producing a 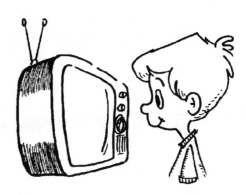 video commercial (television) or designing a printed advertisement (newspaper, magazine, flyer).

Collections

Collect samples of different kinds of advertisements (newspaper, magazine, bulletin board, etc.).

Classroom Guests

Invite someone who is a salesperson or in advertising to visit and tell about his or her job.

Commercial Watch

Watch an appropriate television show that is educational and entertaining. Screen the show for violence, sexism and racism. If you videotape a program, you can view it first to determine its appropriateness. Let children watch the show and tell you when there is a commercial. Talk about what each commercial is advertising.

Commercial Listen

Turn the radio on to a music show and let children move to the music. Tell them to listen for the commercials and stop moving when the commercial starts. Help children identify commercials and what they are advertising.

Traditional Learning Centers

Art

Provide materials to make miniature billboards that could be used in the block area. Billboards could be made by cutting out pictures of products from catalogs or magazines and pasting them on index cards. The cards can be taped to popsicle sticks. Place one stick vertically between two horizontal ones at the bottom and glue.

Blocks

Add billboards to advertise different products in the block area. Explain that billboards go beside the roads.

Housekeeping

Add a transistor radio to the area. Add a video player and television with previewed and recorded television shows and commercials.

Manipulative

Add puzzles and games with pictures of televisions, radios and newspapers.

Science

Add ink pads and stamps.

Resources ●

More information on these resources can be found starting on p. 261.

Books

Anno's Flea Market   *The Trouble with Dad*
Caps for Sale

Songs

When My Shoes Are Loose
   Do You Know

Poems, Rhymes and Fingerplays

Free to Be ... a Family   *Where the Sidewalk Ends*
   Little Abigail and the   *For Sale*
   Beautiful Pony
The Turn of the Tide

9.

Drug Use Prevention

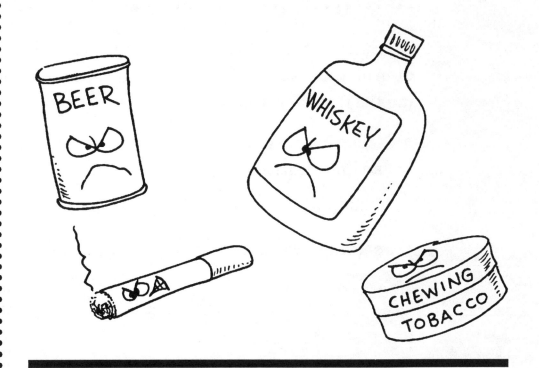

Drug Use Prevention

In this unit, children are introduced to the beneficial and appropriate uses of medicine. Young children usually are not aware of the use of mood modifiers such as opiates, cannabis, amphetamines, barbiturates, hallucinogens, tranquilizers and volatile substances. However, they often are aware of alcohol and tobacco use. Therefore, children should be aware that these substances are not appropriate for children's use and can be dangerous to their health.

Lifestyle Goals

Successful completion of this curriculum will put children on the road to achieving lifelong goals of understanding the importance of:

- following medical recommendations in the use of drugs and medications;

- avoiding the use of potentially harmful drugs;

- obeying laws regarding the use of controlled substances.

Objective 29
When to Take Medicine

Children will be able to explain when it is appropriate to take medicine.

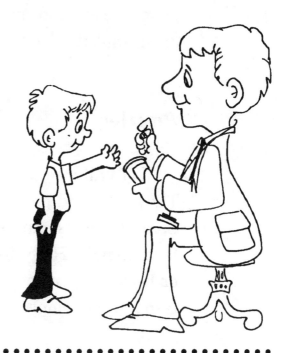

• •

The purpose of this objective is to help children understand that medicine is to help us get well or to prevent illness (immunizations).

Medicine is not candy, and it can make you sick if the wrong kind or amount is taken. Stress again the importance of taking medicine only when given by a responsible person.

Activities

Spinning Wheel

Make a spinning wheel with pictures of people taking medicine, pictures of sick people and pictures of healthy people. Ask children to talk about each picture. Ask children what they see.

Puzzles

Let children look for pictures of people who are sick. They may find pictures of people with crutches or a cast. Some advertisements for headaches and allergies show faces in pain. Help children glue the pictures on cardboard or heavy paper and cut out puzzle pieces. Store in a container or envelope.

Brainstorming

List reasons people take medicine. Expand upon examples of people feeling sick. Let children describe different kinds of illness, such as broken arm, headache, fever, etc.

Collages

Let children make a medicine collage. Encourage children to use pictures of all types of medicines—liquids, pills, sprays, drops, shots, creams, etc.

Field Trips

Visit an animal hospital. Explain that animals get sick and need doctors and medicine, too.

Classroom Guests

Ask a pharmacist to visit and explain his or her job. Ask the guest to talk about the dangers of taking the wrong medicine or too much medicine.

Special Learning Centers

The Medicine Chest

Make a medicine chest to go in a special area. Use silver contact paper on the lid for the mirror. Stock the box with bandages and tape and medicine bottles containing water or cotton.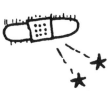

Traditional Learning Centers ....

Art

Add empty medicine containers for children to decorate.

Housekeeping

Add empty medicine containers.

Science

Add empty medicine bottles for children to sort. Provide small pebbles for children to fill the containers.

With close supervision, let children combine:

6 tablespoons salt

6 tablespoons bluing

6 tablespoons water

1 tablespoon ammonia

Mix well and pour slowly over three lumps of soft coal in a pie plate or low bowl. The *garden* takes several hours to grow. Explain that medicine makes things happen to our body just as the contents of the mixture made the garden grow.

Resources ●●

More information on these resources can be found starting on p. 261.

Books

The Dragon and the Doctor
I Wish I Was Sick, Too
Morris Has a Cold

Now One Foot, Now the Other
Samit and the Dragon

Songs

Learning Basic Skills
   Cover Your Mouth

When My Shoes Are Loose
   Legs, Slow Down
   Telephone

Poems, Rhymes and Fingerplays

Finger Frolics
   Stood up Dangerously

Where the Sidewalk Ends
   Band-Aids

Objective 30
Who Should Give Medicine

Children will be able to explain who is appropriate to give medicines (to them).

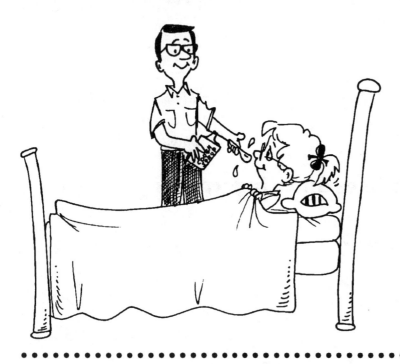

The purpose of this objective is to help children understand that they should be careful from whom they accept medicine.

Medicine is not candy, and it can make you sick if the wrong kind or amount is taken. Stress the importance of taking medicine only when given by a responsible person. Discuss who gives children medicine. This may include doctors, nurses, parents, guardians, babysitters or teachers. Children should *never* take medicine from a stranger or friend without asking their parents first.

Activities ....

Circle Share

Encourage children to talk about times when they took medicine. Ask what the medicine was for and who gave it to them.

Problem Solving

Describe a situation, and ask children what Kevin should do in that situation. Examples: What should Kevin do if...?

- He is sick, and a friend wants to give him a pill to make him feel better.

- He is sick, and his father wants him to take medicine that tastes bad.

- He is sick, and he knows where his medicine is kept. His mother is sleeping, and he doesn't want to wake her up.

Roleplay

Ask children to act like they are playing in their yard and a neighbor tells them to take medicine. What would they do and why? Make up other situations using a friend of theirs, a friend of their parents and a stranger.

Someone Says

In this version, the leader uses his name for every command that is a safe physical activity, such as "Carlos says, 'Jump up and down.'" Every few commands, the leader should say, "Take medicine." Children should follow all the commands except take medicine (because Carlos did not say it). Tell children they should not take medicine unless certain people, such as parents or doctors, tell them to take it.

Permission Form

If you administer medicine in your center, it is highly advisable and required by many state daycare regulations that you have written permission from parents or guardians. If this is the case in your center, show the forms to the children and explain that even teachers cannot decide about medicine for the children. Explain that teachers can give medicine to children in place of the parents or guardians only with their permission. Show children where the parents or guardians have signed.

The Wrong Lotion

Use an 11-inch fashion doll to represent the adult and a smaller doll to represent the child. Make up a story about Mieko being sick and needing medicine. Let her have chicken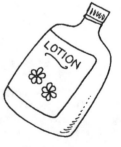

pox. (Explain chicken pox.) Make Mieko scratch and scratch. Let the adult doll put lotion on Mieko's legs. (Really use lotion and cotton and apply to the doll.)

Afterwards, let Mieko itch again and go get the lotion to put on herself. Have the adult doll catch her with the wrong lotion *before* she applies it. The adult doll should explain that the lotion Mieko has is hand lotion and not medicine.

Have the adult doll explain how dangerous it could be to use the wrong medicine and tell Mieko who can give her medicine. Encourage children to ask the people who care for them who is allowed to give them medicine.

Traditional Learning Centers

See suggestions for **When to Take Medicine— Objective 29**.

Resources

More information on these resources can be found starting on p. 261.

Books

I Wish I Was Sick, Too

Songs

When My Shoes Are Loose
  Telephone

Objective 31
Tobacco's Harmful Effects

Children will be able to list some harmful effects of tobacco use.

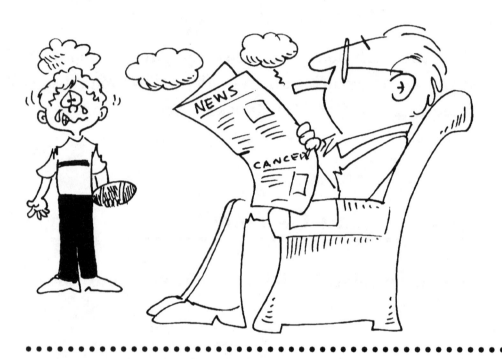

The purpose of this objective is to help children become aware of the harmful effects of tobacco use. Emphasize the effects of smoking, but also include smokeless tobacco (snuff, chewing tobacco) in the discussions. Smokeless tobacco can harm teeth, gums and mouth.

Smoking hurts the lungs and heart, which can slow people down during physical activities like running. Discuss the effects of secondhand smoke (smoke from someone else's cigarette) and how secondhand smoke can hurt people, too. Explain that *secondhand smoke* is the smoke breathed out by a smoker, *sidestream smoke* is the smoke coming from the tip of a burning cigarette.

Cigarettes and other tobacco products cost a lot. A single package of cigarettes may cost $2.00 or more; cigarettes cost a lot of money when you count how much you spend in a week or a month. The money people spend on tobacco could be used to buy other things.

Be careful not to make judgments about people who smoke. Many of the children's family members may smoke. Words such as *bad* can be misunderstood by children. Children are confused when one adult tells them something and another adult gives different or conflicting information. Be sensitive to different views about tobacco use.

Activities

Show Smoke

Ask a smoker to blow cigarette smoke into a clear plastic bottle that has a cotton ball inside. Have children watch to see what happens.

Hard to Breathe

Ask children to hold their breath. Discuss how it feels. Ask children to run either in place or around the playground. Discuss how hard it is to breathe. Explain that it is harder for people who smoke to breathe. Discuss how it feels.

Steam and Smoke

Run or boil hot water until there is steam. Compare steam and smoke. Try to identify pictures through the steam. Discuss the difficulty of seeing through steam and smoke.

Mirror Cloud

Provide a large mirror or several small mirrors for the children. Ask them to breathe out air with their mouths close to the mirror. Encourage children to try to see themselves in the cloudy mirror. Watch to see how long the cloud takes to go away. Clean the mirrors after the activity to discourage the spread of germs.

Walks

Go for a walk and look for the word *hazardous* or words that mean the same thing. Show children the word on cigarette packages. Allow time for discussion.

On a walk, look for No Smoking signs. Discuss where smoking is not allowed (theaters, gas pumps, restaurants, etc.).

Classroom Guests

Ask a health professional (a doctor, nurse or someone from the American Heart Association, American Cancer Society or the American Lung Association) to visit and explain the health problems smoking can cause. Include secondhand smoke in the discussion. Ask the guest to bring pictures or props to help the children understand.

Where Does It Go?

Have pictures of tobacco and cigarettes and nutritious foods. Encourage children to sort the pictures into a box with a smile and the words *Good for You* on it or a box with a frown and the words *Not Good for You* on it.

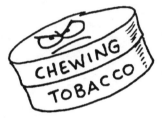

Traditional Learning Centers

Art

Display pictures of fireworks. Explain that fireworks are pretty, but they are hot and can burn us just as cigarettes and cigars can. Let the children make No Smoking signs. Provide many different samples and art materials. Encourage children to design their own creations.

Resources

•••••••••••••••••••••••••••••••••••••

More information on these resources can be found starting on p. 261.

Books

Smokey the Bear

When There Is a Fire, Go Outside

Songs

Free to Be ... a Family
   Jimmy Says

Substance Use Prevention

Children will be able to identify some harmful effects of substance use.

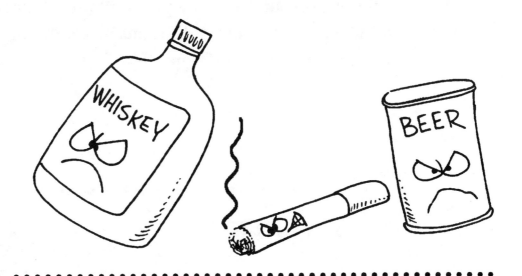

• •

The purpose of this objective is to help children become aware of the harmful effects of using too much of any substance, as well as discourage children's use of any amount of alcohol or other drugs. Explain the meaning of using too much of something as it relates to a variety of topics. For example, too much candy can cause a stomachache.

Unfortunately, some young children see substance use, such as alcoholism or drug addiction, in their own family or living environment. If your students are exposed to such situations, you may wish to use this unit to discuss delicate situations.

One concept that might be appropriate is: Drinking too much alcohol may cause people to lose control. This may result in harm to themselves or someone else. Be careful not to make judgmental remarks about people who drink, since many of the children's family members may drink alcohol.

Words such as *bad* can be misunderstood by children. Children are confused when one adult tells them something and another adult gives different or conflicting information. Be sensitive to different views held by adults regarding alcohol use.

Activities

Where Does It Go?

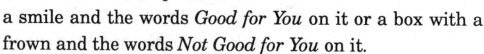

Have pictures of beverages that help your body grow (such as milk or fruit juice) and beverages that do not promote growth (such as soft drinks, coffee, tea or beer). Ask children to sort the pictures into a box with a smile and the words *Good for You* on it or a box with a frown and the words *Not Good for You* on it.

Exercise

Lead an exercise activity that lasts longer than usual. Let children stop when they want to, but ask if they have had too much exercise. Discuss how it feels.

Too Many Toys

Give each child a few small toys such as beads, one-inch cubes or small vehicles. Pass around a container that's too small for all the toys to fit in, and ask each child to put a toy in it.

When the container is full, wait until the children comment. Ask them why all the toys won't fit. The container is too small, and there are too many toys. Have children sort toys and place them back in a container that will hold all the toys.

Roleplay

Ask children to act like they've had too much to eat.

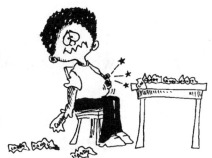

Tell children to act like they've had too much exercise.

Ask children to act like they've had too much to drink (any liquid).

Do You or Don't You?

Explain that some things we do and some things we eat are good for us and help us grow strong and healthy. Other things are not so good for us and may even hurt our body.

Tell children you are going to name some things. The children should decide if each thing is good for them or not so good. If the answer is good for them, children should stand up. List these items: candy, running, beer or wine, sleeping, cigarettes, medicine, shots, etc.

Explain that some people would like to quit smoking but it is very difficult to stop. This may be true for adults who drink alcohol as well.

Traditional Learning Centers

Art

Provide too little paint in each container. Add more when the children notice.

Blocks

Add too many vehicles to fit in the designated area. Rearrange the block building area to be too small until children experience it. Then change it back to the original design.

Housekeeping

Add too many dishes, clothes, etc., to fit in the designated storage place.

Resources ••

More information on these resources can be found starting on p. 261.

Books

Easy Does It
The 500 Hats of Bartholomew Cubbins
Gono and the Magic Hat
It's Too Noisy
My House Is Different

One Day at a Time
The Three Bears
Too Many Animals
Too Many Mittens
Too Much Noise
The Very Hungry Caterpillar

Songs

Free to Be ... a Family
  Jimmy Says
  Yourself Belongs to You

When My Shoes Are Loose
  When My Shoes Are Loose

Poems, Rhymes and Fingerplays

Finger Frolics
  Being Sleepy
  Going to Bed
  Sleepy Head

Where the Sidewalk Ends
  Jimmy Jet and His TV Set

10.

Community Health

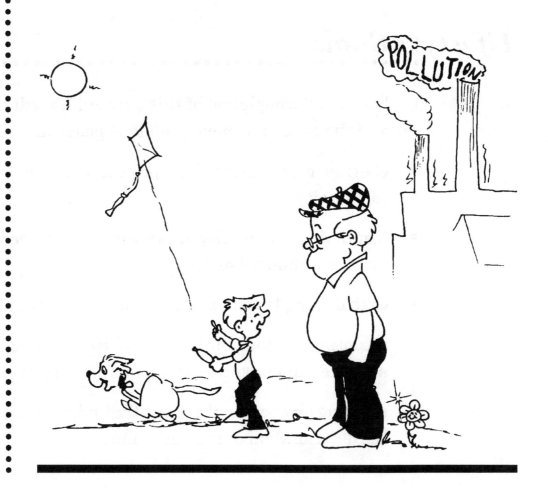

Community Health

In this unit, children are introduced to ways that individuals can help solve community-wide health problems such as environmental pollution, spread of disease and waste disposal. The children will also learn about people, organizations and resources that help community health management.

Lifestyle Goals

Successful completion of this curriculum will put children on the road to achieving lifelong goals of:

- obeying laws designed to protect the health of the community;

- identifying community organizations designed to promote community health;

- contributing to community health programs;

- accepting responsibility as a citizen to support the activities and programs of community health workers;

- avoiding any personal actions that might contribute to the deterioration of the environment.

Here We Go...Watch Me Grow!

Objective 33
Health Helpers

Children will be able to identify people who contribute to good health (health helpers).

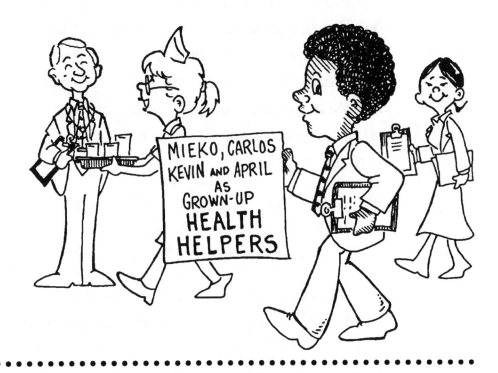

The purpose of this objective is to help children learn the roles of medical, dental and mental health personnel. These professionals contribute to the health and well-being of society as a whole. Children can do their part through preventive health measures, such as dressing appropriately for the weather, staying home and resting when they are sick, etc.

Encourage children to relate their experiences with health professionals. Discuss when it is appropriate to see a doctor, a dentist, a counselor or other community health professional. Discuss where health professionals work (hospitals, health departments, clinics). If your children will be receiving health screening, such as eye exams or hearing tests, discuss the screening procedures before they occur.

Screenings: Medical and dental experiences may be frightening to children, especially if their only experience involves unplanned trips when they are ill or receiving immunizations. We can reduce children's anxiety by helping them become familiar with medical and dental tools, simple medical procedures, health professionals and the screening process.

Screenings are provided by some comprehensive childcare programs, such as Head Start. You need to find out if your program provides screenings.

If your program does not, check with the administration to see if there are any policies that prohibit or discourage screenings being provided through your classroom. If you arrange for screening to occur through the classroom, you should have written permission from parents or guardians.

If policy prohibits arranging a health screening, you may be able to send a note home. The note could encourage family members to arrange screenings for their children. Screenings may be arranged through a family doctor or dentist or through the local health department.

Screenings may be arranged free of charge for your program, especially if your center is nonprofit. Check with local colleges and universities. Nursing students can sometimes provide vision screenings. Speech and communication disorders students may be able to provide hearing screenings. Some health departments provide screenings.

Help children understand that sometimes they see a doctor to find out if they need special help. Discuss the importance of the sense of hearing. Explain that there are ways to help people hear better. Therefore, it is important to know if they can hear well.

Discuss the importance of the eyes and all we can see with them. Explain that if children can't see as well as they should, they can get help. Therefore, they should have their eyes and vision checked.

Activities

Mobiles

As a group, make a mobile of things and pictures of people relating to various health professions. Check a play doctor kit for possible items to use.

Practice Vision Screening

Trace around an adult hand and cut it out. Make enough hands for each child and yourself. Give each child one of the hands. Tell the children to watch your hand and turn theirs to look like yours. While children stand still, move a little farther away and try again (to see if they can still do it at a farther distance). Try it first with the children using both eyes. Then ask the children to cover one eye and try it again.

Blood Pressure

Bring a child's blood pressure cuff to class. Let children practice (with your help) to find out what the cuff feels like when it is inflated. (Do not inflate the cuff very much or leave an inflated cuff on a child more than about 10 seconds.) Let children play with the cuff and stethoscope. They can look for blood vessels in their own and each other's arms, hands, legs and neck.

Pulse

Explain that your pulse and blood pressure tell the doctor what your heart is doing. Have children feel their pulses. The artery in the neck is the easiest to feel. Tell children to place two fingers (not thumb) over their Adam's apple. Next, children pull their fingers slowly to the side of their necks until they feel the thump, thump of their pulse.

Have children run in place for 30 seconds and then feel their pulse. Talk about how much faster it feels.

Let children listen to their pulse with a stethoscope.

Temperature

Show and discuss an outdoor thermometer. Discuss how the doctor or nurse measures people's temperature. Show children various types of thermometers, including digital thermometers and temperature dots. (Dots are laminated circles or strips that are placed on the skin. They change color according to the person's temperature.) Let children take turns putting a temperature dot on their foreheads.

Classroom Guests

If health screenings are provided through your program, invite health professionals who will be part of the children's health screening to visit.

Invite a mental health professional to visit the classroom and talk about his or her job. Explain to children that some people tell the counselor about their feelings.

Brainstorming

Explain that all health helpers have a responsibility (this means it's their job) to help take care of everyone's health. Each person also has the responsibility of taking care of his or her own health. Encourage children to share ideas for taking care of their own health. Examples can include choosing nutritious foods and drinks, exercising, wearing clothes appropriate for the weather, taking medicine when needed and not at any other time, saying no to drugs and alcohol, choosing not to smoke or chew tobacco, etc.

Special Learning Centers

The Eye Doctor

Set up an area for the eye doctor to examine patients. Include an eye chart, doctor's coat and a mirror. Arrange an adjoining area for selling eyeglasses. Provide frames for glasses (remove the lenses) and sunglasses. Place pictures of people wearing glasses around the office.

The Doctor

Set up an area in the classroom for the doctor to examine patients. Include a doctor's coat and a doctor's kit. Include a syringe *without* a needle.

Traditional Learning Centers

Art

Add cotton-tipped swabs to use for painting and in creating collages.

Blocks

Add block accessory dolls representing people who contribute to good health. Add block accessory buildings related to health. Add health-related vehicles.

Housekeeping

Add health profession uniforms.

Manipulative

Add puzzles and games related to health helpers.

Resources •

More information on these resources can be found starting on p. 261.

More information on these resources can be found starting on p. 261.

Books

Dentist
Albert's Toothache
*The Berenstain Bears Visit
   the Dentist*
Come to the Doctor Harry
My Dentist
My Friend the Dentist
When I See My Dentist

Doctor/Hospital
*Curious George Goes to the
   Hospital*
A Drop of Blood
Eric Needs Stitches
A Hospital Story
Madeline
My Doctor

Eye Doctor
Look at Your Eyes

Songs

Circle Around
   The Monster Song

Hug the Earth
   The Family Song

Objective 34
Caring for the Environment

Children will be able to demonstrate ways to help keep classrooms, playgrounds and homes both clean and safe.

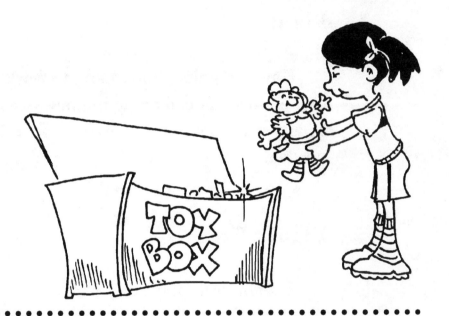

The purpose of this objective is to help children realize that keeping the environment clean is everyone's responsibility. Refer to resource books on how to save the environment. They have interesting and useful information to share with children.

The cleanliness of the areas in which people live affects their health and safety. While adults have the general responsibility to keep the environment clean, children can learn good helping habits that they will still practice as adults. Explore ways that children can help.

Remember that modeling the behavior you want from children makes a big impact. Look for ways to help children learn to take care of their environment in everyday activities.

Activities

Fix It

Have a regular time when you work with children to fix broken toys instead of buying new ones. Let children help in any way they can. Invite skilled volunteers to help as needed.

Plant a Tree

Let children plant and care for a tree. Help them see that their tree will provide a home for birds, shade to other animals and beauty for people. Explain that the tree also helps clean the air.

Trash Cans

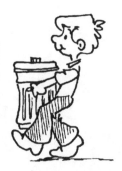

Bring a variety of clean trash cans to the classroom. Encourage children to examine and compare the various kinds of containers. Look at pictures of other types of containers.

Collections

Collect newspapers or aluminum cans for recycling. Then take a trip to deliver the materials to the closest recycling center (or have the center pick them up). Help children understand that trees are cut down to make paper.

Traditional Learning Centers

Art

Design the center so children can use it independently and clean up after themselves. If running water is not available, include water and sponges.

Blocks

Add a gas and service station, so the vehicles can be checked for safety. Add a highway department and people to work there. Tell children the people need to inspect the roads.

Housekeeping

Add cleaning instruments and supplies, such as a vacuum cleaner that really works, a broom, a mop, dusting cloths, etc.

Resources ●

More information on these resources can be found starting on p. 261.

Books

Joshua's Day   *The Little Red Hen*

Songs

Free to Be ... a Family   *Peace Is the World Smiling*
  On My Pond   *Hug the Earth*
Hug the Earth   *Whale Gulch Rap*
  Garbage Blues   *When My Shoes Are Loose*
  Super Kids   *Legs, Slow Down*
Learning Basic Skills   *Pick It Up*
  Safe Way

Poems, Rhymes and Fingerplays

Free to Be ... a Family   *Sarah Cynthia Sylvia Stout*
  On My Pond   *Would Not Take the*
Where the Sidewalk Ends   *Garbage Out*
  Helping   *Tree House*

Resources

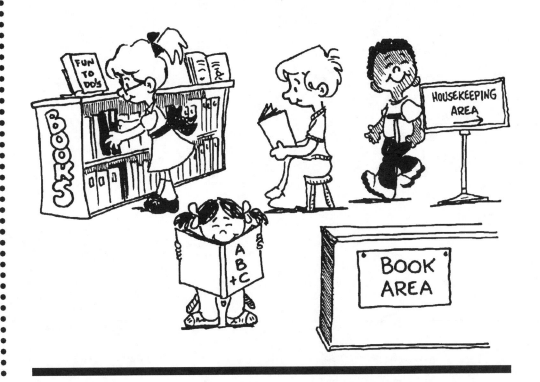

Here We Go, Watch Me Grow!

Book List

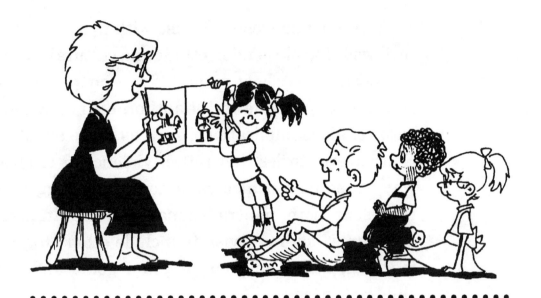

During story time choose short books with large pages and many colorful pictures to read with the entire class. Small pages and more detailed pictures are generally better for one or two children to look at or listen to at a time. Also, stories in which the children can participate hold their attention longer. Such stories either ask questions, give directions for movement, or have rhymes or repetition for children to chant.

Encourage children to participate in story time. You

may also use attention-getters such as flannel boards, puppets or dressing up to tell the story.

Before reading or telling stories, become familiar with the book. Then be sure that you and the children are seated comfortably and all the children can see and hear you. Learn to hold the book so you can read and show the picture, or establish a pattern with the children so they know you will show them the picture after you read the page.

The books suggested for use with this curriculum were reviewed to avoid gender, ethnic and cultural stereotyping. In an effort to show respect for each person's right to personal religious views, the authors did not include stories with religious implications, such as those about holidays. Neither are stories that reflect violence or cruelty in any way. An effort was also made to include suggestions that represent both nontraditional and traditional family structures. You may wish to include other stories in your teaching, based on your program goals and individual children's needs.

The book lists that accompany each objective include many award-winning books that relate to health as well as to other areas. You don't have to use all the suggestions. Select the books you feel your children will most enjoy. Some books are listed with more than one objective.

The following book list includes all the books recommended in this curriculum. The books are listed alphabetically by title, with authors' and publishers' names. Suggested book titles are listed alphabetically with each objective.

Abby
Caines
Harper & Row, New York

ABC-ing an Action Alphabet
Beller
Crown, New York

About Dying: An Open Family Book for Parents and Children Together
Stein
Walker, New York

Albert's Toothache
Williams
Dutton, New York

Alexander and the Terrible, Horrible, No Good, Very Bad Day
Viorst
Macmillan, New York

All Alone with Daddy
Fassler
Behavioral Publications, New York

All Kinds of Families
Simon
Albert Whitman, Niles, IL

The Alligator's Toothache
Covan
Lothrop, Lee & Shepard Books, New York

Anno's Flea Market
Anno
Philomel Books, New York

Apple Pie and Onions
Caseley
Greenwillow Books, New York

Are You My Mother?
Eastman
Random House, New York

Ask Mr. Bear
Flack
Macmillan, New York

Automobiles for Mice
Ets
Viking, New York

A Bargain for Frances
Hoban
Harper & Row, New York

Be a Frog, a Bird or a Tree: Carr's Creative Yoga Exercises for Children
Carr
Doubleday, New York

The Berenstain Bears Visit The Dentist
Berenstain
Random House, New York

The Biggest Nose
Caple
Houghton Mifflin, Boston

Big Sister and Little Sister
Zolotow
Harper & Row, New York

Bill and Pete
  de Paola
  G. P. Putnam's Sons, New York

A Bird Can Fly
  Florian
  Greenwillow Books, New York

Black Is Brown Is Tan
  Adoff
  Harper & Row, New York

Blueberries for Sal
  McCloskey
  Viking, New York

Blue Bug to the Rescue
  Poulet
  Children's Press, Chicago

The Boy Who Cried Wolf
  Evans
  Albert Whitman, Niles, IL

Boys and Girls, Girls and Boys
  Merriman
  Holt, Rinehart & Winston, New
    York

Bread and Jam for Frances
  Hoban
  Trophy, New York

Brown Bear, Brown Bear, What Do You See?
  Martin
  Holt, Rinehart & Winston, New
    York

Bunnies and Their Sports
  Carlson
  Viking Kestrel, New York

Button in Her Ear
  Litchfield
  Albert Whitman, Niles, IL

Calico Cat's Exercise Book
  Charles
  Children's Press, Chicago

Caps for Sale
  Slobodkina
  Scholastic, New York

The Carrot Seed
  Krauss
  Harper & Row, New York

Chicken Little
  Burgess
  Harrison House, Tulsa

Clifford, the Small Red Puppy
  Bridwell
  Scholastic, New York

Clifford's Good Deeds
  Bridwell
  Four Winds Press, New York

Chilly Stomach
  Caines
  Harper & Row, New York

Come to the Doctor Harry
  Chalmers
  Harper & Row, New York

Cornelius
  Lionni
  Pantheon Books, New York

Crafty Chameleon
  Hadithi
  Little, Brown, Boston

CROSS
  McCracken and Holt
  National Assication for the Education of Young Children, Washington, DC

Curious George Goes to the Hospital
  Rey
  Scholastic, New York

Curious George Takes a Job
  Rey
  Scholastic, New York

Daydreamers
  Feelings & Greenfield
  Dial Books, New York

The Dead Bird
  Brown
  Harper & Row, New York

Do You Know What I'll Do?
  Zolotow
  Harper & Row, New York

The Dragon and the Doctor
  Danish
  Feminist Press at the City University of New York

A Drop of Blood
  Showers
  Thomas Y. Crowell, New York

Drummer Hoff
  Emberly
  Prentice-Hall, Englewood Cliffs, NJ

The Ear Book
  Perkins
  Random House, New York

Easy Does It
  Hallinan
  Hazelden, Center City, MN

Eric Needs Stitches
  Marino
  J. B. Lippincott, Philadelphia

Everett Anderson's Friend
  Clifton
  Holt, Rinehart & Winston, New York

Everett Anderson's Goodbye
  Clifton
  Henry Holt, New York

Everybody Takes Turns
  Corey
  Albert Whitman, Niles, IL

Eye Book
  Le Sieg
  Random House, New York

Fat, Fat Calico Cat
  Charles
  Children's Press, Chicago

A Father Like That
  Zolotow
  Harper & Row, New York

Fire! Fire! Said Mrs. McGuire
  Martin
  Holt, Rinehart & Winston,
    Canada

First Delights
  Tudor
  G. P. Putnam's Sons, New York

The 500 Hats of Bartholomew Cubbins
  Dr. Seuss
  Scholastic, New York

Free to Be ... a Family
  Thomas & Friends
  Bantam Books, New York

Friday Night Is Papa's Night
  Sonneborn
  Puffin, New York

The Giraffe Who Got in a Knot
  Brush & Geraghty
  Price Stern Sloan, Los Angeles

Girls Can Be Anything
  Klein
  Dutton, New York

The Giving Tree
  Silverstein
  Harper & Row, New York

Gilberto and the Wind
  Ets
  Viking, New York

Gono and the Magic Hat
  Currier
  Wellin World, Old Greenwich,
    CT

Gooseberries to Oranges
  Cohen
  Lothrop, Lee & Shepard Books,
    New York

Grandma's Wheelchair
  Heniod
  Albert Whitman, Niles, IL

Grandpa
  Borack
  Harper & Row, New York

Green Eggs and Ham
  Dr. Seuss
  Random House, New York

Growing Story
  Krauss
  Harper & Row, New York

Grownups Cry Too
  Hazen
  Lollipop Power, Carrboro, NC

Grumbel, the Fire-Breathing Dragon
    Fleishman
    Harvey House, New York

Happy, Healthy Pooh Book
    Disney
    Golden Books, New York

Harry, the Dirty Dog
    Zion
    Harper & Row, New York

The Hating Book
    Zolotow
    Harper & Row, New York

Hold My Hand
    Zolotow
    Harper & Row, New York

A Hole Is to Dig
    Krauss
    Scholastic, New York

A Hospital Story
    Stein
    Walker, New York

Howie Helps Himself
    Fassler
    Albert Whitman, Niles, IL

How Many Teeth?
    Showers
    Thomas Y. Crowell, New York

How You Were Born
    Cole
    Morrow Junior Books, New York

Human Body Book
    McGuire
    Platt & Munk, New York

The Hunter and the Animals
    de Paola
    Holiday House, New York

I Can Be a Truck Driver
    Behrens
    Children's Press, Chicago

I Can, Can You?
    Parish
    Greenwillow Books, New York

I Can't Wait
    Crary
    Parenting Press, Seattle

I Have Feelings
    Berger
    Behavioral Publications, New
        York

I Know an Old Lady
    classic
    Bantam Books, New York

I Know I'm Myself Because
    Greenberg
    Human Sciences Press, New
        York

I'm Mad at You
  Gikow
  Muppet Press

In The Forest
  Ets
  Viking, New York

Ira Sleeps Over
  Waber
  Houghton Mifflin, Boston

Is That Your Sister?
  Bunin & Bunin
  Pantheon Books, New York

It Looked Like Spilt Milk
  Shaw
  Harper & Row, New York

It's Too Noisy
  Cole
  Thomas Y. Crowell, New York

I Want It
  Crary
  Parenting Press, Seattle

I Wish I Was Sick, Too
  Brandenberg
  Greenwillow Books, New York

Jenny Lives with Eric and Martin
  Bosche
  Gay Men's Press, London

Jo, Flo and Yolanda
  De Poix
  Lollipop Power, Carrboro, NC

Joshua's Day
  Surowiecki
  Lollipop Power, Carrboro, NC

Just Like Me
  Ets
  Viking, New York

Just Us Women
  Caines
  Harper & Row, New York

Kevin's Grandma
  Williams
  Dutton, New York

Leo the Late Bloomer
  Krauss
  Thomas Y. Crowell, New York

Let's Be Enemies
  Udry
  Harper & Row, New York

Let's Eat
  Fujikawa
  Zokeisha, Japan

Like Me
  Brightman
  Little, Brown, Boston

A Little Book of Love
  Anglund
  Random House, New York

Little Rabbit's Loose Tooth
  Bate
  Crown, New York

The Little Red Hen
  Galdone
  Houghton Mifflin, Boston

Little Witch's Big Night
  Hautzig
  Random House, New York

The Longest Journey in the World
  Morris
  Holt, Rinehart & Winston, New
    York

Look at Your Eyes
  Showers
  Thomas Y. Crowell, New York

Look at You
  Daly
  Golden Books, New York

Lots of Mommies
  Severance
  Lollipop Power, Carrboro, NC

*Loudmouth George and the Big
Race*
  Carlson
  Carolrhoda Books, Minneapolis

Love You Forever
  Munsch
  Firefly Books, Willowdale,
    Ontario, Canada

Madeline
  Bemelmans
  Viking, New York

Make Way for Ducklings
  McCloskey
  Puffin, New York

Martin's Father
  Eichler
  Lollipop Power, Carrboro, NC

May I?
  Riehecky
  Children's Press, Chicago

May I Visit?
  Zolotow
  Harper & Row, New York

Messy Bessey's Closet
  McKissack
  Children's Press, Chicago

*Mom and Dad Don't Live Together
Anymore*
  Stinson
  Firefly Books, Scarborough,
    Ontario, Canada

Mom Is Single
  Paris
  Children's Press, Chicago

Mommy Works on Dresses
  DeGrosbois, et al.
  Women's Press, Toronto

Moon Man
  Ungerer
  Harper & Row, New York

Morris Has a Cold
   Wiseman
   Dodd, Mead, New York

Mothers Can Do Anything
   Lasker
   Albert Whitman, Niles, IL

Moving Day
   Tobias
   Random House, New York

Mr. Grumpy's Motor Car
   Burningham
   Thomas Y. Crowell, New York

Mr. Grumpy's Outing
   Burningham
   Holt, Rinehart & Winston, New
      York

My Daddy Is a Nurse
   Wandro
   Addison-Wesley, Reading, MA

My Dad Takes Care of Me
   Quinlan
   Annick Press, Willowdale,
      Ontario, Canada

My Dentist
   Rockwell
   Greenwillow Books, New York

My Doctor
   Rockwell
   Macmillan, New York

My Favorite Place
   Sargent & Wirt
   Abingdon Press, New York

My Five Senses
   Aliki
   Thomas Y. Crowell, New York

My Friend the Dentist
   Watson
   Golden Books, New York

My Grandpa Died Today
   Fassler
   Human Sciences Press, New
      York

My Grandson Lew
   Zolotow
   Harper & Row, New York

My House Is Different
   Hallinan
   Hazelden, Center City, MN

My Mom Travels a Lot
   Bauer
   Frederick Warner

*My Mother and I Are Growing
Strong*
   Maury
   New Seeds Press, Berkeley, CA

My Mother Lost Her Job Today
   Delton
   Albert Whitman, Niles, IL

My Mother the Mail Carrier
Maury
Feminist Press at the City University of New York

My Name Is Not Dummy
Crary
Parenting Press, Seattle

New Life: New Room
Jordan
Crowell, New York

No Measles, No Mumps for Me
Showers
Harper & Row, New York

Now One Foot, Now the Other
de Paola
G. P. Putnam's Sons, New York

One Day at a Time
Hallinan
Hazelden, Center City, MN

On Mother's Lap
Scott
McGraw-Hill, New York

Our Teacher's in a Wheelchair
Powers
Albert Whitman, Niles, IL

Our Tooth Story: A Tale of Twenty-two Teeth
Kessler
Dodd, Mead, New York

Pat the Bunny
Kumhardt
Golden Books, New York

People
Spier
Doubleday, New York

Peter's Chair
Keats
Harper & Row, New York

Play It Safe
Webb
Golden Books, New York

Play with Me
Ets
Viking, New York

The Quarreling Book
Zolotow
Harper & Row, New York

Rosie and Roo
Greenberg
Growth Program Press

Safe Sally Seatbelt and the Magic Click
Gobbel & Laster
Children's Press, Chicago

Samit and the Dragon
Currier
Wellin World, Old Greenwich, CT

See What I Can Do: A Book of
Creative Movement
Boray
Prentice-Hall, Englewood Cliffs,
NJ

The Sheep Book
Goodyear
Lollipop Power, Carrboro, NC

Sheila Rae, the Brave
Henkes
Greenwillow Books, New York

She's Not My Real Mother
Vigna
Albert Whitman, Niles, IL

Smokey the Bear
classic

The Snowman
McKee
Lothrop, Lee & Shepard Books,
New York

The Snowy Day
Keats
Viking, New York

Something Is Wrong at My House
Davis
Parenting Press, Seattle

Spring Is Here
Parker
Row, Peterson

Stephanie and the Coyote
Crowder
Upper Strata, Bernalillo, NM

Stone Soup
Brown
Charles Scribner's Sons, New
York

Stopping by Woods on a Snowy
Evening
Frost
Dutton, New York

Stories for Free Children
Pogrebin
McGraw-Hill, New York

The Story of Ferdinand
Leaf
Viking, New York

Strangers
Chlad
Children's Press, Chicago

Sunshine
Ormerod
Lothrop, Lee & Sheppard Books,
New York

The Surprise Party
Hutchins
Macmillan, New York

Sweetie, A Sugar Coated
Nightmare
Currier
Wellin World, Old Greenwich, CT

The Sweet Touch
  Balian
  Abingdon Press, New York

Swimmy
  Lionni
  Alfred A. Knopf, New York

Talking Without Words
  Ets
  Viking, New York

Teeth
  Ricketts
  Grossett & Dunlap, New York

Ten Apples up on Top
  Le Sieg
  Random House, New York

Ten, Nine, Eight
  Bang
  Greenwillow Books, New York

*The Tenth Good Thing About
Barney*
  Viorst
  Atheneum, New York

That New Baby
  Stein
  Walker, New York

There's a Nightmare in My Closet
  Mayer
  Dial Books, New York

The Three Bears
  classic

Tight Times
  Hazen
  Penguin, New York

Tommy Takes a Bath
  Wolde
  Houghton Mifflin, Boston

Too Many Animals
  Ipcar
  Scholastic, New York

Too Many Mittens
  Slobodkin
  Vanguard Press, New York

Too Much Noise
  McGovern
  Houghton Mifflin, Boston

The Train
  Welber
  Pantheon Books, New York

A Tree Is Nice
  Udry
  Harper & Row, New York

The Trouble with Dad
  Cole
  G.P. Putnam's Sons, New York

The Trouble with Mom
  Cole
  Coward-McCann, New York

The Twins Strike Back
  Flournoy
  Dial Books, New York

Two Good Friends
Delton
Crown, New York

The Ugly Duckling
Andersen
Scholastic, New York

The Velveteen Rabbit
Williams
Platt & Munk, New York

The Very Hungry Caterpillar
Carle
Philomel Books, New York

Watch out for the Chicken Feet in Your Soup
Paola
Prentice-Hall, Englewood Cliffs, NJ

Wellin Magic
Currier
Wellin World, Old Greenwich, CT

What Spot?
Bonsall
Harper & Row, New York

When I Cross the Street
Chlad
Children's Press, Chicago

When I Ride in a Car
Chlad
Children's Press, Chicago

When I See My Dentist
Kuklin
Bradbury Press, New York

When There Is a Fire, Go Outside
Chlad
Children's Press, Chicago

Where Is Daddy?
Goff
Beacon Press, Boston

Where the Wild Things Are
Sendak
Harper & Row, New York

Why Am I Different?
Simon
Albert Whitman, Niles, IL

William's Doll
Zolotow
Harper & Row, New York

Will I Have a Friend?
Cohen
Macmillan, New York

Will It Be Okay?
Dragonwagon
Harper & Row, New York

Wind Rose
Dragonwagon
Harper & Row, New York

Yertle the Turtle and Other Stories
   Dr. Seuss
   Random House, New York

Yoga for Children
   Harvey & Richards
   Bobbs-Merrill, Indianapolis

You Are Special
   Currier
   Wellin World, Old Greenwich, CT

You Look Ridiculous
   Waber
   Houghton Mifflin, Boston

Your Family, My Family
   Drescher
   Walker, New York

Song List

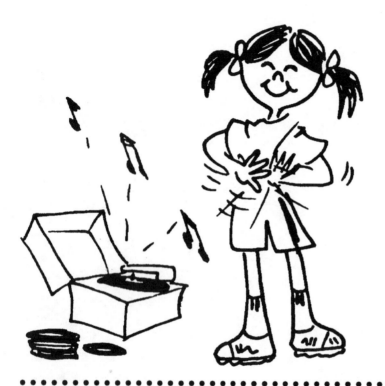

Songs can be enjoyed by children in different ways. Children can listen to, move to, play instruments with and sing songs. Singing is probably the most common way to use songs, but it's the most difficult to teach and supervise.

Short songs with simple tunes and motions are easiest for young children to learn. Before teaching a song to children, use it first as background for the rhythm band, moving or motions.

When teaching children a song, first sing it and play it all the way through to give them an overall idea of the song.

Give children a reason for listening to the song. For example: You can tell the children to listen to the song and stand up every time they hear a specific word such as *happy*. You also can explain that you want them to listen so they can sing with you later. Be creative and invent different reasons for children to listen.

Next, try singing one line to the children, and then have them sing it back to you or with you. Use pictures or motions to help children remember the words to the song. Continue to teach the song line by line until the children have learned the entire song. Children will probably need more than one session to learn the entire song. Before teaching them another song, be sure that the children feel comfortable with the one they just learned.

The songs suggested for use with this curriculum were reviewed to avoid gender, ethnic and cultural stereotyping. In an effort to show respect for each person's right to personal religious views, the authors did not include songs with religious implications, such as holiday songs.

Songs that reflect violence or cruelty in any way are not included. An effort was also made to include suggestions that represent both nontraditional and traditional family structures.

The records from which individual songs are suggested may include other songs that do not meet these criteria. However, you may wish to include these and other songs in your teaching, based on your program goals and individual children's needs.

A list of recommended songs is included with each objective. Select the songs that you and your children will most enjoy. Remember, it is important to use the same song in a variety of ways, so it becomes familiar to children but does not get old. Try singing a song loudly, softly, happily, sadly, quickly, slowly, without some of the words or with new words. Try humming it, tapping it or clapping it.

The following list includes all the records from which the songs suggested for each objective were taken and their respective artists and publishers. Recommended songs are listed by record title with each objective.

The following records or tapes are resources from which the suggested songs are taken.

All of Us Will Shine
  Tickle Tune Typhoon
  Tickle Tune Typhoon, Seattle

And One and Two
  Ella Jenkins
  Folkways Records and Service,
    New York

Baby Beluga
  Raffi
  Troubadour Records, Willowdale,
    Ontario, Canada

Circle Around
  Tickle Tune Typhoon
  Tickle Tune Typhoon, Seattle

Everything Grows
  Raffi
  Troubadour Records, Willowdale,
    Ontario, Canada

Free to Be ... a Family
  Marlo Thomas & Friends
  A & M Records, Hollywood, CA

Hug the Earth
  Tickle Tune Typhoon
  Tickle Tune Typhoon, Seattle

*Learning Basic Skills (Through
Music, Vol. III)*
  Hap Palmer
  Educational Activities, Freeport,
    NY

One Light, One Sun
  Raffi
  Troubadour Records, Willowdale,
    Ontario, Canada

Peace Is the World Smiling
  (various)
  Music for Little People, Redway,
    CA

*Singable Songs (for the Very
Young)*
  Raffi
  Troubadour Records, Willowdale,
    Ontario, Canada

Sing Your Sillies Out
  Wolf Trap
  Wolf Trap Foundation, Vienna,
    VA

Teaching Peace
  Red Grammer
  Smiling Atcha Music, Peekskill,
    NY

Travellin' with Ella Jenkins
  Ella Jenkins
  Folkways Records and Service,
    New York

Voyage for Dreamers
  Pamela Ballingham
  Mother Earth Productions,
    Tucson, AZ

When My Shoes Are Loose
  Billy B
  Do Dreams, Takoma Park, MD

Poem, Rhyme and Fingerplay List

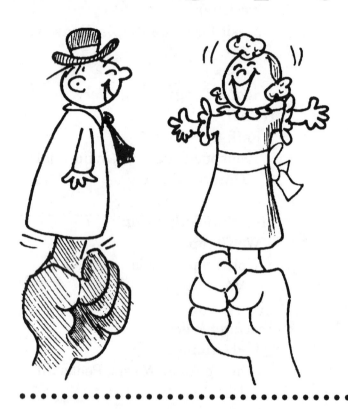

For a good balance of activities, poems, nursery rhymes and fingerplays can be read to the children.

When reading these aloud, show children the action as you say the words all the way from beginning to end. Give children a purpose for listening to you. Repeat the motions and words, asking children to participate in the motions.

Depending on the length of the fingerplays, you may need to encourage children to join in on the first line, key words or rhyming words along with the actions until they have learned them. Provide various times during the day for children to practice. Transition times are especially good for this. Be sure that children feel comfortable with the poem, nursery rhyme or fingerplay before teaching a new one.

The poems, rhymes and fingerplays suggested for use with this curriculum were reviewed to avoid gender, ethnic and cultural stereotyping. In an effort to show respect for each person's right to personal religious views, the authors did not include works with religious implications, such as those relating to holidays. Neither did the authors include poems, rhymes or fingerplays that reflect violence or cruelty in any way. An effort was also made to include suggestions that represent both nontraditional and traditional family structures.

The books from which individual poems, rhymes or fingerplays are suggested may include other materials that do not meet these criteria. However, you may wish to include some of these works and others in your teaching, based on your program goals and individual children's needs.

Many suggestions are listed with the objectives. It is not required that you use every one. Select those you and your children will enjoy most.

The following books are those from which the suggested poems, rhymes and fingerplays are taken, followed by their respective authors and publishers.

Resources

Finger Frolics (revised 1983)
Cromwell, Hibner, Faitel
Gryphon House, Mt. Rainier, MD

Free to Be ... a Family
Thomas & Friends
Bantam Books, New York

Where the Sidewalk Ends
Silverstein
Harper & Row, New York

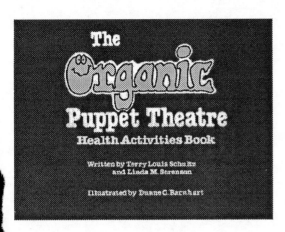
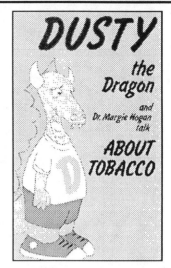
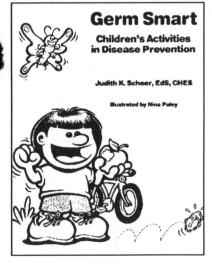
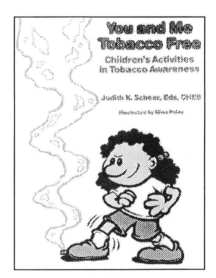